BEFORE
PHARMACEUTICALS

BEFORE PHARMACEUTICALS

EMOTIONAL HEALING WITH CHINESE MEDICINE

WILL FUDEMAN, LAc, LCSW

BRYCE
CULLEN
PUBLISHING

**BRYCE
CULLEN
PUBLISHING**

PO Box 731
Alpine, NJ 07620
brycecullen.com

ISBN 978-1-935752-29-5

Library of Congress Control Number: 2012948033

Printed in the United States of America

10 9 8 7 6 5 4 3 2 1

"Chinese medicine has for me been the fulfillment of a search for a congenial system of healing that embodies the inseparability of body and mind, spirit and matter, nature and man, philosophy and reality. It is a personal, subtle, gentle, yet highly technical medical system, which allows me to be close to essence- to the life force- both my own and that of others. The reasons for using it, teaching it, and discussing it are twofold. First, it works. Second, it is a masterpiece of harmony, intricacy, and movement, which never ceases to engage me, fascinate me, and intrigue me. It surrounds me like nature, or a great work of art."

—Leon Hammer, MD, *Dragon Rises, Red Bird Flies: Psychology and Chinese Medicine*

CONTENTS

Foreword

BY THEA ELIJAH, LAC

"What the practitioner of Chinese medicine is looking to find are ways to release the person from the constraints that have held her back from expressing her genuine, heartfelt truth."

—Will Fudeman

Will Fudeman is a teacher of the fearless compassion that is necessary to get to the root of a problem--be it on a personal, social or global level. Our current reliance on psychiatric drugs as a primary approach to treating mental and emotional disorders is a problem that requires a willingness to think and feel beyond the scope of easy answers.

That's because easy answers are--well, easy. But they are often not satisfying answers. To find truly healing solutions, we need courage to confront the complex and interconnected reality of our situation, which often initially gives rise to a lot more questions than answers. This can be daunting; it can feel discouraging and overwhelming enough that we might be tempted to stick with the easy answers, even knowing that they are not really answers.

The ability to consider problems on the level of complexity necessary to attempt a truly comprehensive healing response requires the willingness to face the discomfort of not having immediate answers that will fit neatly into our existing paradigm. We need to have compassion and caring, but also a stalwart ability to dare to consider beyond the familiar, in order to discover not just one root for our problems, but the vast interconnected network of roots, and what might be needed to shift the situation as a whole. Often this requires a much broader scope of inquiry, but surprisingly, as when a familiar landscape is seen from a distance, this broader view can make obvious the patterns and possibilities that were hidden from us before.

Pharmaceutical solutions to mental or emotional problems target the biochemistry of individuals as the focal point of their intervention. *Before Pharmaceuticals* looks at individual emotional suffering in a wider context-- in the context of the individual as a whole (body mind and spirit), and in the context of the world in which we live. Specifically, *Before Pharmaceuticals* avails us of the healing paradigm of Chinese medicine and its approach to healing mental and emotional problems.

Chinese medicine is much more than a system of healing physical illnesses. It is a deeply rooted (and continuously evolving) worldview that is capable of encompassing every aspect of human life. The combination of this ancient medicine and Will's contemporary training and experience as a social worker, and his many decades of political activism, combine in this book to allow for a comprehensive look at the necessities and potentialities of emotional healing that does not shirk the level of complexity required to deliver an implementable paradigm shift. Better yet, Will Fudeman has done the hard work for us; his years of experience allow him to express this much needed vision of alternative care for emotional health issues as a very readable, easily grasped synthesis of how to apply ancient Chinese healing principles in our lives today.

Maybe there are some easy answers after all--found in the simple traditional wisdom of listening to our body, listening to our lives, and returning to methods that have been practiced by humans striving to be in harmony with their world for thousands of years.

Even if neither you nor anyone close to you is taking pharmaceutical drugs for emotional issues, this is a book worth reading, because it is about practical tools and resources for emotional health (and healing) in a world where suffering is not necessarily a sign of illness. We all have, at times, cause for fear, anger, or grief; we may have experienced events which were shocking or traumatic. How do we respond, as whole beings? If, in the midst of our lives, we have found our emotions overwhelming, where can we turn for help?

Before Pharmaceuticals gives us a vision of life in which strong emotions, and even emotional distress, are not something to be afraid of. They are an opportunity to engage with our lives, and more importantly to engage with ourselves, such that we can bring to our lives a clearer and more heartfelt expression of our selfhood. Instead of being overwhelmed by our emotions, we can use them as doorways to self-discovery, and as the source of our most true and enduring response to our world today.

Will Fudeman (and the other authors who have been invited to contribute to this book: Stephen Cowan, Heiner Fruehauf and myself) speak at length about the nature of the Heart in Chinese medicine, not only as a physical organ but as the steady, clear center of consciousness in each person. The common phrases "losing heart" or "taking heart" bespeak this sense of the Heart as a place inside of ourselves which is beyond momentary mood or thought, a place of awareness and sovereignty within ourselves. In times of strong emotion, what makes all the difference in the world is whether we are overwhelmed, or whether we are able to allow ourselves to feel all that we truly feel within a sense of ourselves as connected to the steady and sovereign awareness of the Heart.

If so, this does not mean that life will suddenly be easy. We will still have pain and suffering. Nothing in this book promises otherwise. What is offered here is a practical orientation towards living with Heart at the center of our emotional response to life, connected with the rhythms of nature and the world as a whole. This allows us to feel and move through life events with a sense of meaning and purpose that carries us through the pain, through the disruptions, on a journey of creation and discovery: no matter what life brings us, our task is bringing our truest and most heartfelt selves to life.

Beginnings

The first person ever to receive hands-on healing from me was my father. Dad would return home from a long day's work, lay down on the living room rug, and ask me to massage his back and shoulders. He gave me appreciative feedback, and instructions: "A little lower to the left; oh, yeah..." As I kneaded his muscles, feeling his breathing change with the pressure of my thumbs, I instinctively knew, even as a young child, that I was doing something useful.

Dad also introduced me to traditional forms of healing that were not mainstream in upstate New York. He regularly took me and my brother to Kaufman's Health Club (known simply as 'the Schvitz',) where he brought us into the Finnish steam room, and showed us how to do the traditional eastern European *pleytze* form of massage with a brush made of oak leaves, dipped in soapy water. Sweating in the steam room, sprawled on a wooden bench, the brush of oak leaves swirling around and pressing into my back was an experience that I knew my father enjoyed, which he shared with me. I didn't know anything about acupuncture needles or moxibustion, but I knew that unusual tools from distant lands could enhance our quality of life here in the

United States.

My father understood the value of living a balanced life. He worked hard, and he encouraged me to recognize the importance of recreation, which he said helped to 're-create' any person who had been working long and hard hours. My dad's common sense interest in activities that enhanced his feeling of well-being served to nourish the seeds of my interest in learning about healing.

I first experienced an urgent need for healing after being in an accident when I was 26 years old. Sitting in my car at a red light on Jewett Parkway in Buffalo, New York in January of 1977, I felt a sudden explosive shock as a Chevrolet slammed into the rear end of my VW Rabbit. My glasses flew off my face with powerful force as my body was thrust into the seat belt, then slammed back into the seat. I found my way out of that car, walked to a friend's house nearby, my back in terrible pain, which persisted for months afterwards. I received chiropractic treatments from a practitioner in the neighborhood that didn't help me very much, as I continued to tighten up in pain, driving to work on icy roads for the rest of that winter. By the following fall, I began making plans to move to a milder climate in northern California, where I hoped I might find someone to help me heal. It was that car crash in Buffalo that led to my discovery of the world of Chinese medicine.

A friend I saw in a natural foods Store in Fairfax, California told me about an acupuncturist who had learned Chinese medicine by apprenticeship with a healer on Taiwan. I met Michael Broffman at his home, where he spent more than an hour talking with me. That first time I saw him, Michael felt my pulse, and then asked me, "Do you have a tendency to get in relationships with women about 10 years older than you?" Since the longest-lived relationship in my life to that point had been with a woman nine years older than me, I wondered how he came up with that question. He said something about my Liver pulse and my Kidney pulse. I decided to continue to see him since his approach to thinking about health was based on something new and interesting to me.

When the pain in my back got worse a few months later, going down my leg with an intensity that made it uncomfortable to sit down, Michael gave me my first acupuncture treatment. I was amazed and pleased to experience that terrible pain easing and diminishing as it moved down my leg and out of my body.

Over the 12 years that I saw Michael regularly, I learned to practice *Tai Chi* and *Qi Gong*, shiatsu massage, and to think differently about food. I was working part-time at a county-funded agency as a psychotherapist, interacting daily with other psychotherapists. When a friend from my shiatsu class began acupuncture school in San Francisco, I wondered how difficult it would be to memorize all the point locations.

A few months after my father died, fifteen years after I met Michael Broffman, I decided to go to acupuncture school. I inherited some money from Dad, so I suddenly had the opportunity to change the course of my life. I decided the best thing I could do was to learn skills that could benefit other people in the sorts of ways I had benefited from my relationship with Michael. I was surprised at how many people thought it was a great idea, including my mother!

Attending the New England School of Acupuncture (NESA) was something like Harry Potter and his young wizard friends attending Hogwarts. There were all sorts of teachers with unique gifts, introducing their students to a powerful world of healing. And, these teachers were each unique human beings, with quirky personalities, great strengths, and occasionally, human failings. I remember how odd it seemed to me to see two of my teachers smoking cigarettes in the parking lot between classes. Each of them did what they could to help us learn techniques of diagnosis and treatment from practitioners in the long lineage of healers from east Asia. Every day, we had the opportunity to treat one another and see how quickly our discomforts or pains or moods of the day could be transformed.

Five years after my father died, my mother had surgery for a cancer remarkably similar to the cancer that killed Dad. After having a huge section of her gastrointestinal tract removed, she complained to her doctor of a reduced appetite. Her oncologist prescribed an SSRI antidepressant, which catalyzed unprecedented panic, high anxiety, severe insomnia and suicidal ideation. The family mobilized support to keep her safe, I found her a competent psychiatrist to help her taper off the drug, and after a hellish six weeks, my mother seemed to return to her old self. After witnessing first-hand the moment-by-moment impact of a bad reaction to a psychiatric drug in my family, it's not surprising that I developed an interest in alternative approaches to treating emotional imbalances.

My mother lived with cancer, which metastasized to her lungs, and then her brain, for another five years. When I visited her, she would often ask me to treat her with acupuncture soon after my arrival. The acupuncture treatments would alleviate her symptoms (the cough, the pain, the dizziness). Spending quiet time together as she relaxed with the needles frequently set the tone for a good visit. I felt grateful to have a skill which helped my mother feel more comfortable during the difficult months of her illness.

When practicing the *Zhi Neng Qi Gong* form, as the hands pass over the kidneys, we thank our parents for the essential vitality we received from them when we were born. I like to picture my parents' faces as I practice the slow, meditative movements that help me to feel the life force flowing through me. I feel fortunate to have the opportunity to share practices and perspectives I've learned that can bring healing and appreciation to the lives of others.

1

BEFORE PHARMACEUTICALS

*P*sychiatry in the 21st century treats all sorts of emotional and mental problems with pharmaceutical drugs. These drugs offer short-term alleviation of symptoms to some of the people who take them, while other people who take psychiatric drugs find that their symptoms get worse. Many people who take antidepressants say they notice no effect whatsoever. Marcia Angell, MD (1), Robert Whitaker (2), Christopher Lane (3) and others offer powerful criticisms of psychiatry's reliance on these psychiatric drugs, and the real harm they can cause. Chinese medicine offers one alternative to pharmaceutical treatment that has a very long history of effectiveness in healing imbalances that arise from what the Chinese refer to as negative emotions. For thousands of years before pharmaceuticals, Chinese medicine has offered treatments and practices to harmonize the emotions.

People who find pharmaceutical medication helpful in alleviating symptoms of anxiety or depression still might want to read this book because Chinese medicine's strategies can provide a path to living more joyfully in the body, and might help anyone experience a fuller life. Many people who take pharmaceuticals would prefer not to experience the side effects, and might want to transition to an alternative approach before the drugs become less effective or lead to an exacerbation of symptoms. Eventually, people can discover a safe path to letting go of psychiatric medications (under their doctor's supervision).

Learning about Healing, Chinese style

During my first rotation in Student Clinic at the New England School of Acupuncture, a gray-haired woman with a chronic dry cough came for treatment. When she returned the week after her first acupuncture experience, she asked me, "What did you do? All week long, I've been relaxed and almost cheerful while still living with my mother, who usually drives me up a wall. What is this acupuncture doing? It's like I'm a different person!" What I did was try to alleviate her chronic dry cough. Her experience of greater ease in dealing with a difficult living situation made clear to me that treatment with acupuncture could have a positive (unintended) impact on emotions.

My Chinese medicine textbooks told of combinations of acupuncture points and Chinese herbal formulas to treat depression, anxiety, insomnia, and mania. As a psychiatric social worker with experience working in mental hospitals, community mental health centers, and residential treatment centers, I wondered *how* treatment with Chinese medicine might be helpful to people suffering from emotional problems. The words in the textbooks, while they sounded poetic, didn't explain *how* these needles and herbs could 'calm the spirit', 'nourish Heart *yin*', or 'smooth Liver *Qi*'. After practicing Chinese medicine for fifteen years, my experiences have given me some notions of how emotional healing happens. When people describe their symptoms and ask if acupuncture can help them, I suggest that it's worth trying. A large percentage of the people who come to me for acupuncture say to me, as they are leaving my office after the first treatment: "Thanks a lot- I feel better". Readers of this book can discover how people might feel better from these treatments with needles that seem so foreign to most of us who grew up in a western culture dominated by allopathic medicine and its pharmaceutical drugs. You can also discover how *qi gong* (meditative physical exercises which promote a healthier attitude toward life) could be practices you might enjoy making part of your daily routine.

Some of the *qi gong* practices I do every morning were created thousands of years ago. Designed by Taoist masters to enable practitioners to create feelings of harmony, aliveness, and connection to all of nature, *qi gong* can provide such experiences today. Chinese herbal formulas and acupuncture treatments to calm the spirit have also been used for thousands of years, before pharmaceutical treatment for depression and anxiety came into common practice. If Western medical practitioners routinely referred people struggling with anxiety or depression to an acupuncturist or *qi gong* instructor before prescribing psychiatric drugs, many of them could experience greater well-being and relief of discomfort, as well as learning skills in self-regulation of mood.

Practitioners of Chinese medicine in Western cultures have learned a very different way of thinking about health, the human body, and life than the Western science that gave birth to modern allopathic medicine.

The Chinese believe that there are three basic factors that might (sometimes in combination) cause disease: external pathogenic influences, inherited deficiencies (making one prone to certain types of disease), and internally generated illnesses-- caused by an unbalanced emotional life. Rather than focus on a particular virus or bacterium as a cause, the Chinese think about the whole person. The emotional and the physical are naturally intertwined.

Regardless of a person's Western diagnosis- Rheumatoid Arthritis, Bipolar disorder, or Migraine headaches- the practitioner of Chinese medicine takes the pulse, looks at the tongue, asks questions, and observes the person to ascertain what is the relative balance or imbalance of *Qi*, Blood, *Yin*, and *Yang*. Are there deficiencies, or excessive accumulations? Is the person too hot or too cold? Is the problem superficial or deep within the person? Treatment has the purpose of catalyzing an energetic shift toward greater harmony and balance. An extremely effective treatment will resonate with a person's deepest virtues, and bring forth strength of character. It might be fair to assert that such a treatment heals on a level deeper than Prozac.

Specifically, sometimes an acupuncture treatment can

shift an unhealthy attitude. A woman was referred to me by her psychotherapist because she was so distraught over being left by her husband that she could not imagine ever emerging from her anxious depression. Her therapist hoped that acupuncture might provide a catalyst to shift this woman's dark and hopeless mood.

When this woman found herself laughing on the treatment table during her second acupuncture treatment, she was astounded. "How can I be laughing? I'm terribly depressed!" That treatment did not permanently 'cure' this woman's depression, but it gave her an experience of joy and freedom and the possibility of change, even in the midst of her hopelessness. It could have been a turning point in her sense of what could be possible for her. She continued to see me for acupuncture for about six months, recognizing that the treatments could lift her spirits. She joked that she wished she could just stay in my office because she felt so good there. But, when she finally accepted the fact that her husband was not coming back to her, she decided to discontinue both acupuncture and her psychotherapy, asserting that she didn't want to feel better. She told me that she was sick of all her friends advising her to "move on". She didn't want to "move on"; she wanted to "go back to how it was before". She had the idea that her misery would serve as just punishment to her husband for betraying her. I'd learned approaches to take with acupuncture and Chinese herbs to help heal a Heart injured by betrayal, but as with most genuine forms of emotional healing, they don't offer a "quick fix". If and when she decides to reconsider the possible benefits of the "feeling better" and "moving on" approach, this woman might come back for more treatment and more therapy. Most of us don't like to hold on to bitterness forever, and most of us appreciate feeling better from emotional suffering if we can find a path that works for us.

I now see Chinese medicine as an ideal complement to psychotherapy for many mild to moderate emotional problems, and preferable to Western pharmaceuticals in most cases that are not extremely severe. To the extent that disturbing emotions experienced for a long period of time (months or years duration) lead to chronic emotional states of anxiety, depression, frustration or anger, Chinese medicine's interventions are ideally suited to heal the hurt by catalyzing an energetic shift toward balance, and a healthy attitude.

Gifted practitioners of Chinese medicine in the West bring their unique life experiences to the work they do. Years of studying techniques of diagnosis and treatment and the philosophy of Chinese medicine combine with the unique perspective of each practitioner, so that the healing experience one might have with one acupuncturist is not exactly the same as the healing experience the same person might have with another acupuncturist. Some acupuncturists focus primarily on physical complaints, and alleviating discomfort. Some acupuncturists think more creatively about healing, and give their clients insights into the Chinese approach to 'living a Proper Life'. You may seek acupuncture primarily for relief of physical complaints. Or- if you've suffered from low self esteem or depression or anxiety for years, you may be open to discovering a more satisfying way of life for yourself.

In this book, I write about my experiences treating people with serious emotional problems. I begin with my experiences as a psychotherapist, and continue by telling about my experiences treating people with a combination of Chinese medicine and some form of psychotherapy, either with me, or with another licensed professional. I describe other aspects of living that can be healing for anyone wanting a more balanced emotional life, including Chinese forms of meditative movement like *tai chi* and *qi gong*, various forms of creative expression, and active participation in efforts to make one's community (or world) a better place. I tell about one client whose treatment with me was not enough for her to recover from her emotional problems, and I finish with a chapter about ways that Chinese medicine can serve a deeply healing role near the end of life.

****

I graduated from the New England School of Acupuncture in May of 1997, and began my practice of Chinese medicine when I received my license in September of that year. I've sought out more experienced teachers and colleagues to help guide me to learn more about what Chinese medicine can do for the people who come to me, and some of my favorite teachers have written articles that are included as appendices at the end of this book. Each of their experiences brought them to understandings of healing that are best expressed in their own words, and I feel honored to have the opportunity to introduce my readers to their work.

I studied the "Spirit of the Herbs", from a Five Element perspective, with Thea Elijah, L.Ac., former director of Herbal Medicine at the Academy of Five Element Acupuncture. I find Elijah's teachings fascinating and clinically useful.

I've transcribed two sections of a lecture on the Five Virtues (which Thea has edited for clarity) to create the essays found in Appendix C. I picked the sections on Water (transformation from Fear to Wisdom) and Wood (transformation from Anger and Frustration to Visionary Creativity) because the issues addressed by these elements apply most obviously to the treatment of anxiety, depression, and post-traumatic stress disorder. For readers interested in Thea's teaching on the virtues of the other three elements (Fire, Earth, and Metal), the lectures on these elements are available for free at www.perennialmedicine.com under 'Audio Downloads'-"The Five Virtues".

Several of my teachers, including Ted Kaptchuk, Thea Elijah, and Bill Mueller, have made the point that Traditional Chinese Medicine (or T.C.M.) as it is taught in most acupuncture schools in America and in mainland China today lacks the spiritual and emotional dimensions that had traditionally been inherent in the medicine. After the Communists took over ruling China in 1949, they influenced their schools of TCM to focus on the physical body rather than the spirit or the emotions. For example, Elijah teaches that the herbal formula *Du Huo Ji Sheng Tang* had originally been designed for "the pain of attachment to transient phenomena." Under the Communists, and at many acupuncture schools in America like NESA, we learn that the formula is for arthritis pain in the joints. I became interested in learning more about the aspects of traditional Chinese medicine that had been discarded by the Communists.

Heiner Fruehauf, founding professor at the School of Classical Chinese Medicine in Portland, Oregon, is a scholar as well as a gifted clinician who I first heard speak at the "Building Bridges of Integration" conference in October of 2008. Dr. Fruehauf's essay "All Disease Comes from the Heart: The Pivotal Role of the Emotions in Classical Chinese Medicine" (Appendix B) cites classical Chinese writings such as the *Neijing*, or *Yellow Emperor's Classic of Medicine,* to reveal that early Chinese healing focused on the emotions. Dr. Fruehauf quotes Liu Zhou, a 6th century philosopher: "If the spirit is at peace, the heart is in harmony; when the heart is in harmony, the body is whole; if the spirit becomes aggravated, the heart wavers, and when the heart wavers the spirit becomes injured; if one seeks to heal the physical body, therefore, one needs to regulate the spirit first". (Fruehauf, Appendix B, p. 103)

When I heard Dr. Fruehauf quote these sources in a keynote lecture at Building Bridges, I felt excited. My acupuncture school didn't require or even encourage us to read these classic sources. It was Thea Elijah who sparked my interest in the lost spiritual and emotional aspects of Chinese medicine, and Heiner Fruehauf who made clear to me that emotional healing was a central aspect of Chinese medicine, not merely one type of symptom that acupuncture could help alleviate.

According to many teachers and practitioners, the most respected healers look at the quality of the *shen* coming through a person's eyes and are able to use traditional diagnostic tools (including pulse and tongue diagnosis) to discern specific disharmonies arising from troubled emotions that may lead to physical illness if not treated. From the *Neijing*: "The superior physician makes it his prerogative to treat disease when it has not yet structurally manifested, and prevents being in the position of having to treat disorders that have already progressed to the realm of the physical". (Fruehauf, Appendix B, p. 104).

For readers interested in a deep and well-documented look at the classical sources of emotional healing in Chinese medicine, Dr. Fruehauf's essay is an excellent introduction. Its concluding section focuses on "the power of ritual" and the emotional therapy system of Wang Fengyi, a Confucian educator of the 19th and 20th centuries. Wang Fengyi's system of healing involved storytelling that was able to "turn the heart of the patient... literally talking the disease away by appealing to one's higher nature." (Appendix B, p. 117) Dr. Fruehauf has traveled to China in recent years to spend time with healers of Wang Fengyi's lineage, and directly "...witness the intense process of storytelling and ensuing physical cleansing" that is reputed to completely cure serious diseases, including "...diabetes, congenital heart disease and many types of cancer". (Appendix B,

p. 118) For more of Dr. Fruehauf's work, the website www. classicalchinesemedicine.org offers other articles, and video resources.

Dr. Stephen Cowan, MD, FAAP, a pediatrician and Five Element acupuncturist, asserts that healthy children provide a model for us about living in harmony with nature. Dr. Cowan describes his notion of the "basic sanity" of self-regulation as a gift that we adults can learn from children in his essay "Healing Emotions in Children". (Appendix A) The merging of Dr. Cowan's experience as a pediatrician working with children with his deep grounding in Chinese philosophy give his teaching and writing a unique and re-freshing perspective. His book *Fire Child, Water Child* (c. 2012, New Harbinger) offers guidance to parents in under-standing the five types of ADHD, so that they can improve the self-esteem and attention of their children.

Please enjoy delving into each of the Appendices at any time during your reading of *Before Pharmaceuticals*. These teachers have enriched my understanding of emotional healing with Chinese medicine, and I trust their writings can touch you deeply as well.

2

CHARACTER OF THE HEALER AND QUALITY OF THE HEALING RELATIONSHIP

During the years I worked in Community Mental Health agencies (in Buffalo, NY, and then in northern California), I was exposed to a variety of approaches to psychotherapy. My first job after receiving my MSW was as a Crisis Counselor, where I was encouraged to help my clients focus on achievable goals that might be "accomplished" in 10 sessions. Some of my clients had serious chronic problems that did not fit this crisis model, and my supervisor allowed me to continue seeing a few clients who were just beginning to make some progress after the tenth session. My supervisor recognized that these clients could benefit from having an ongoing relationship with a caring young therapist who wanted to be supportive of their growth.

By the time I began working at my second agency job, the county Human Services Center where I was hired in northern California, I had a few years of that crisis model informing my way of working with people. Basically, I tried to help the client identify achievable goals they wanted to work on in therapy. When a nice but vaguely dissatisfied potter named Harold didn't have any specific goals or issues to work on with me, I wondered, after about a year of counseling, what was the point of the treatment. Did he want to work on his marital relationship? What did he want to change? He told me he enjoyed my company. But, what he really wanted to do was to be the sort of person who could approach a fully set formal dinner table, and with a flick of his wrist, pull out the tablecloth and leave everything on the table standing. Our sessions together didn't seem to be getting him any closer to realizing anything like this fantasy. Rather, we sat as he complained about how unappreciated he felt being a potter in California, and how little money he was making. He said that in Japan, he would be deeply respected for his craftsmanship.

I let Harold know that I couldn't imagine how sitting with me was going to help him make more money or bring more esteem to potters in the United States. While I appreciated that he enjoyed my company, I felt that he needed something to give him a push toward change and growth, rather than more months of sitting with me, feeling stuck. I suggested that Harold and I choose a date to be our final session, and encouraged him to come up with a way to spend our final time together that he felt would be a good way to say goodbye.

My supervisor thought I was wrong to 'fire' Harold. He thought that sitting with Harold's vague discomfort was the essence of therapy. Maybe. But, I didn't feel that Harold was getting where he wanted to go by sitting with me talking about his same ongoing discontents. What Harold had been telling me was that he wanted to make some kind of dramatic movement that would make him beam with a sense of accomplishing something difficult.

Harold decided to take me to a wild rocky beach about 15 miles south from the community where he lived to teach me about ocean fishing for our final "session". I can recall the powerful surf, the salt spray, and Harold casting his fishing rod. Within a month, Harold and his wife (a Japanese woman) moved to Japan, where he was in fact able to make much more money, and was regarded more highly as a master potter. Close to a year later, Harold turned up in the center of town, glowing, thanking me for all I had done for him. He handed me his card, encouraging me to visit him in Japan, where he was feeling much happier. It was as if he had pulled out that tablecloth, and was amazed and delighted at what he'd been able to do.

According to my supervisor, what I'd done wasn't therapy. Maybe not. But, Harold was grateful to me for the time we'd shared, and for shaking something up that allowed him to make his dramatic move.

While I was working at that Human Service agency near the Pacific Ocean, I was seeing the acupuncturist Michael Broffman fairly regularly for guidance, and when needed, for healing. Occasionally, I would stop by his clinic on Pine Street and have a chance encounter with Michael. In a brief moment, Michael would greet me and smile, and

I would experience an energetic shift- toward vitality, lightness, and benevolent thoughts. There was something about my relationship with Michael that was different from what I felt toward any therapist I'd ever known. I wanted to offer something to my clients like what Michael offered to me.

Heiner Fruehauf tells of the "transmission" from the healer - achieved by an "uncompromised lifestyle of virtuous conduct" which is the catalyst of a powerful healing response. This focus on healing coming from transmission brings to mind the power of what Carl Rogers described as an attitude of "unconditional positive regard." A gifted therapist may demonstrate brilliant analytic insights or clever paradoxical interventions, but the client's experience of relief and growing sense of self-esteem seems to stem more from the felt sense of being in the presence of caring, benevolent attention than anything specific that the therapist *does*.

Healthy personalities develop in the presence of the caring attention of one's parents, grandparents and the other adults seen as guides and sources of wisdom. Inadequate parenting, broken families, and a culture where figures of authority (such as parents, teachers, and priests) prove to be flawed and seriously lacking seems to lead to a society with many individuals in need of healing.

Chinese diagnostic techniques (pulse and tongue diagnosis, or abdominal palpation) provide guidance to the practitioner about what strategies might be likely to catalyze an energetic shift toward balance and health. It may be true that an elegant treatment with needles and an herbal formula that helps restore balance in a person experiencing distress can be delivered by a practitioner who scarcely speaks the language of his or her client. Still, regardless of herbs prescribed, needles inserted, or *Qi Gong* exercises recommended, it seems to be the essence of the relationship between the person and the healer that allows for deep healing. (See *A General Theory of Love* by Lewis, Amini, and Lannon for an explanation of the brain science of 'limbic resonance' which provides a plausible way to understand how this actually happens.) (4)

The Chinese approach may utilize tools that seem foreign to most Americans, but the basic attitude of the healer is consistent with the basic attitude of an effective counselor or therapist. The person who has been deprived of caring attention in their childhood is likely to benefit from relationships that provide caring attention (whether the activities that take place in the healing relationship focus on energetic intervention with needles, herbs, and touch, or on insights about family dynamics) to maximize the likelihood of genuine healing of deficits or traumatic wounds.

Lewis, Amini and Lannon assert that emotional healing in psychotherapy takes years, and despite various modern techniques promising effective brief therapy, genuine changes in how a person experiences their emotional world usually requires long-term treatment. Chinese medicine's approach to emotional healing could catalyze more rapid changes in the troubled mind, but the evidence that this takes place is mostly anecdotal. An acupuncture treatment that 'nourishes the Heart' or 'moves stagnant Liver Qi' seems to catalyze what months of a therapist's empathetic listening to the expression of a client's repressed anger allows to develop: a person who feels more free to experience himself or herself as worthy of being cared for and heard. To date, there are few studies of the efficacy of acupuncture for emotional concerns like depression. A 2012 study published in the Canadian Journal of Psychiatry ...

"... investigating the efficacy of acupuncture as a monotherapy for major depressive disorder (MDD) and as a tool to augment the effects of antidepressants (AD) drugs suggests that acupuncture may be a safe and effective treatment in both these regards....However, the body of evidence based on well-designed studies is limited, and further investigation is called for." (5)

For those who are open to hearing anecdotes from individuals telling about what changed their lives, many people I know could describe the role acupuncture has played in catalyzing their emotional healing.

Given that Chinese medicine developed in a society qualitatively very different from the western scientific society that most readers of this book live in, it is difficult to prove that particular treatments help with particular diagnostic conditions. Chinese diagnostics provide complex and individualized insights into each person's constitution and relative state of imbalance. A treatment that could be successful in alleviating one person's headache might have little effect on another person's pain, depending on what combination of factors cause the headaches. Is the headache caused by 'deficiency' or caused by an 'excess' condition? It's fair to say something similar about alleviating one person's depression; it's possible that choosing to needle certain acupuncture points or prescribing a particular herbal formula could greatly help one person, while accomplishing very little for someone else. What's contributing to the depression? Frustration over many years? Exhaustion at lack of success in one's chosen vocation? Loss of relationships? The Chinese medicine practitioner would treat several people suffering from depression, caused by various different situations, in very different ways. The pulse and tongue of the people would likely show different imbalances, and lead the practitioner to make choices consistent with the unique diagnostic signs.

The world-view of Chinese medicine provides an energetic perspective that values flowing movement over stagnation, and pays attention to the natural rhythms of the seasons and the phase of a person's life. Most people I know who regularly see an acupuncturist (either myself or a colleague) report a quality they value in their connection with the acupuncturist as a healer, as well as the experience of the treatment. For many, acupuncture and some of the practices and values of Chinese medicine serve as an ideal complement to psychotherapy- more balancing and grounding than psychiatric drugs.

Effective therapeutic relationships (whether with a psychotherapist or with an acupuncturist) require that the practitioner pay careful attention to what the client says and to what the client communicates by his or her way of being. The different professions provide different templates of how to understand what we notice in a person. Where a psychotherapist might be seeing evidence of a personality disorder, an acupuncturist might see a person with a Wood constitution with *"Qi* Constraint" and "Liver *Yang* Rising." In either case, the person is more complex than the diagnosis, and the skilled practitioner's choices of how to develop a relationship can be more important than a particular insight or intervention.

The role of the healer in Chinese medicine is more like a friendly model of how to live a "proper life" than the classic psychotherapeutic "blank slate" that the client will develop a transference toward, illuminating the client's relations with his or her parents. The acupuncturist may offer specific suggestions about healthy choices in activities, foods, and even how to enjoy free time- all of which will be intended to help bring the person's life into a more harmonious balance. If a person has gone through a serious emotional breakdown and has been prescribed psychiatric drugs, the acupuncturist will still give treatments intended to re-establish a healthy balance. The Chinese medicine practitioner will often recommend or teach skills and approaches (such as *Qi Gong*, aerobic exercise, or yoga) that might make it easier for the person to manage challenging emotions. Once the client develops habits and practices that empower him or her to feel more balanced, he or she often decides to ask for their prescribing physician's help in tapering off and discontinuing their medications.

Focusing on Virtues rather than Pathology

As a freshman student in a Psychology 101 class at Cornell University, I remember reading a study analyzing the role of teachers' expectations of their students' performance in school. Teachers who expected their students to do poorly had students who did poorly, while teachers who expected good performance had students who did well.

As a second year Social Work Student at SUNY at Buffalo, I attended a weekly Case Conference at the University Health Service where I'd been placed for my internship. Each week, counselors would describe a client they were doing their best to help, and each week, the MD Psychiatrist on staff would explain why one could not expect 'this person' to be able to participate in any satisfying relationships, why one could not expect 'that person' to be able to achieve any success in the career of their choice, and each week, I sat there silently wondering, "How does he know what the future can hold for these people?" Recalling the study I'd read for Psych 101 eight years before, I wondered how many therapists with low expectations for their clients' future growth might have been limiting the depth of healing possible for their clients in working with them.

In Thea Elijah's teaching, based on neo-Confucian texts, the practitioner approaches the possibilities for any client in a treatment relationship in a very different way from that psychiatrist in Buffalo in 1976. In Appendix C, Thea focuses on two of the Five Virtues, and explains how Five Element practitioners can become skilled at perceiving how a person would look when they were healthy (even if they are currently suffering from multiple pathologies). If that article on teacher expectations applies to healers' expectations, one might expect that treatment with Five Element acupuncturists could be qualitatively different from treatment with MD psychiatrists. Of course, a gifted psychiatrist like Milton Erickson was also able to see the health beyond the client's pathology. Erickson's teaching tales offer delightful examples of trusting in the person's unconscious abilities to heal. (6)

For some people, taking a pharmaceutical can help him or her cope with emotional challenges more effectively, whereas treatment with acupuncture might help release long-standing trauma held in the body, and open up new possibilities for growth. There are dozens of approaches to psychotherapy, and each of them can help people. Some therapists develop gifts in helping to catalyze emotional healing, while other therapists might help a person deal with a situation without reaching the essence of the problem or even aiming at any sort of transformation, subtle or profound. The Chinese medicine practitioners who look for the virtue that is the other side of the pathological coin have an advantage in bringing out the best in their clients.

A troubled person who is motivated to learn how to become a more self-assured and competent person with a better sense of humor and a better ability to empathize with others is more likely to grow in that direction than a person who sees himself or herself as a hopeless case. A person with serious emotional problems will be likely to develop an attitude toward possibilities for growth close to the attitude of his or her primary practitioner. A psychotherapist who cannot see the healthy person living inside the troubled person displaying pathological behavior is less likely to catalyze healthy change. It helps a great deal to have some notion of what we might expect to see in a healthier manifestation of this individual so that we can recognize what progress toward that goal looks like.

3

DOING THE DISHES AND PLAYING VOLLEYBALL:
TREATMENT OF A CHRONICALLY ANXIOUS AND DEPRESSED WOMAN

A 40 year old woman, Molly, came to see me for treatment for depression. She complained, with a desperate urgency, of horrible thoughts, difficulty sleeping, and feeling physically unattractive and uncomfortable with her overweight body. She was taking her third pharmaceutical antidepressant, and told me she had not experienced any benefit from any of them, or from her therapy at the county Mental Health Clinic. She told me that Prozac and Paxil had given her terrible PMS symptoms, while on Effexor, she was "crying all the time". She also took an anti-anxiety medication, which could calm her down for about a half hour, but tended to leave her feeling even more desperate as the drug began to wear off. Molly had quit her career, and was now unemployed, living alone in a house that she described as a mess.

Molly was articulate, engaging, and liked to smile and

laugh. She was able to connect with warmth. These are not the typical attributes of a person suffering from depression, and I saw them as strengths that would help in her healing. She told me she had extremely low self-esteem, which she associated with her critical mother. (Her father had died when she was 16 years old). She came to see me twice weekly because she found that acupuncture could transform her mood from a confused and desperate hopelessness to a feeling that she was okay being herself.

During the first several months she came for treatment, she felt in a precarious state, experiencing emotions she described as "jagged". Encounters with friends or conversations with her mother could put her into a dramatic, despairing mood. Bad news or a difficult interaction could bring on a negative feeling, and her fear of experiencing these negative feelings seemed to spiral out of control, as she would judge herself for feeling badly. She chose to spend most of her time alone, except for her visits with me, her acupuncturist and counselor.

As a licensed social worker, I was able to offer counseling to Molly as well as acupuncture and Chinese herbs. We would sit and talk during the first part of her session, and then she would go to the treatment table for acupuncture, where I would needle points to calm the Spirit, nourish Heart and Kidney *Yin*, and move constrained Liver *Qi*, depending on what her pulse, tongue and situation suggested on each visit.

Her racing thoughts would slow down as her body relaxed with the needles in place. After a treatment, she found she could be calm enough to focus on achievable goals. She would have a more realistic perspective, which would allow her to think more clearly about what actions she might take to address any situation she might be in, whether involving her relationships with family members, men in her life, or potential employers or friends.

I became familiar with patterns of behavior that reinforced Molly's low self-esteem, and I encouraged her to make healthy changes. After a few months in treatment, Molly took a part-time job (despite her fears that she couldn't tolerate working). She also decided to stop using marijuana. She found it very difficult to get herself to exercise, stop eating 'junk food', or to stop spending time with people who treated her badly .

A typical session with Molly would begin with her describing to me a disturbing experience she had gone through since our last meeting. An ex-boyfriend would treat her badly, a friend would be in crisis, her mother would call her and say things that got her feeling guilty and very angry. I would listen, make a common sense suggestion about an action she might take to avoid getting even more upset, and then Molly would be ready for acupuncture. She would leave in a cheerful mood, and return in a few days in the middle of another intensely emotional upset

After she reverted to smoking marijuana and quit her job, I felt that working with me alone wasn't providing all the support Molly needed. I strongly encouraged her to go to a therapist other than me (and I referred her to a colleague), and I recommended she continue to see me for acupuncture. She followed this suggestion, with good results.

Molly began to turn her life around. She found two part time jobs she felt good about, and was able to stay away from smoking marijuana. She began to act in a more self-caring way in relation to both her mother and men she was dating. She began to report making healthy choices, and feeling good about those choices. She would beam as she described the progress she had made washing a sink full of dishes. After avoiding participating in group sports for years, Molly reported that she joined in a community volleyball game- which had once been her favorite sport. She was able to enjoy the game, rather than focusing on ways she might not be 'good enough' (because of her overweight body or her lack of adequate skill).

After two years of regular acupuncture, Molly felt solid enough in herself to stop treatment. It's hard to say what allowed her to recognize that sometimes we feel sad and that's a natural part of life, not an indication of a flawed character with no hope of improvement. I imagine that somehow, the combination of her relationship with me and with her therapist, and the acupuncture and herbs led to what she experienced as genuine healing. Molly told me, "It's like I have your voice in my head. When I start getting upset, I hear this calm voice of Will suggesting that I slow down and look at what I can actually do to make things better. And, it works!"

She sent me a card expressing her gratitude:

"I just wanted to thank you from the bottom of my heart.

I don't know how long it will last but I do know I couldn't have gotten here without you."

I called Molly to ask her permission to write about our work together. She was delighted to hear from me, and felt pleased to have me write about her experience. She said, "You saved my life! And don't forget to mention how horrible the pharmaceuticals were for me- all four of them."

It's probably fair for me to say that my perspective on psychiatric drugs is colored by the fact that many of the people who come to me for treatment are people who have unsatisfactory experiences with them. People who respond positively to Prozac or Zoloft, and are not very troubled by side-effects, are less likely to seek Chinese medicine to help treat their depression or anxiety. Still, according to studies referred to by Robert Whitaker (author of *Anatomy of an Epidemic: Magic Bullets, Psychiatric Drugs, and the Astonishing Rise of Mental Illness in America),* in an interview with Jed Lipiniski: 'It should be understood that they're not fixing any chemical imbalances...I think they should be used in a selective, cautious manner. And honestly, they should be used on a short-term basis." (7) The information and thinking in Whitaker's book and in the writings of Z'ev Rosenberg, L.Ac. (chair of the Herbal Studies Program at Pacific College of Oriental Medicine) might encourage even people who have had success with SSRI medications for years to consider tapering off the drugs, and making use of Chinese medicine to help make the transition smoother. (Rosenberg, Z'ev, "A Chinese Look at Western Pharmaceuticals") http://www.acupuncture.com/herbs/pharma.htm)

The intention of treatment with acupuncture and Chinese herbs is to restore harmony and balance where there has been disharmony and imbalance. To the extent that toxic or abusive relationships cause the imbalance, nurturing and healing relationships are likely to be at least as significant a restorative as acupuncture treatments and herbs. The work I did with Molly was more than acupuncture. I met her with the 'unconditional positive regard' that Carl Rogers described as essential to the therapeutic relationship. I paid attention to the sort of tone that would be likely to open Molly to the possibility of change. With Molly, humor was a powerful mood-altering strategy. One of her strengths was her ability to laugh, which allowed her to lighten her judgments of herself.

This is not to say that she stopped having strong feelings. Rather, she learned (as Ram Dass/Richard Alpert once said): "I still have the same neuroses as I had 20 years ago; I've just learned to be more compassionate with myself." Instead of panicking at the onset of a powerful emotion, Molly learned to notice the experience of the emotion, and make choices about what to do about the emotion and the experience or the person which triggered that emotion. Her sense of herself has transformed. She originally sought help because she saw herself as a "depressed person." Now she experiences herself as a person, like other people, with feelings and issues to deal with as she lives her life.

After decades of feeling the victim of abusive, uncaring relationships, Molly learned to practice having awareness of her own needs, asking for what she wanted, and making choices about what to do based on whether others are willing to acknowledge and be responsive to her needs and wants. She has chosen to have relationships with people who are truly supportive friends to her, and to minimize her contact with people who treat her badly.

4

TREATING THE HEART—THE PHYSICAL ORGAN AND THE EMOTIONAL CENTER OF CONSCIOUSNESS

What causes a heart attack, or other forms of heart disease? We might think about the role of diet (too much animal fat clogging the arteries), we can think about the role of cigarette smoking or a family history of heart disease. And, when we know a person who has had a heart attack, we might think of how that person deals with the stress in his or her life. We might not be very surprised when a person who works a very stressful job, then comes home to a family situation that seems in constant crisis, suffers a heart attack.

Jake originally came to me to treat an outbreak of shingles about 12 years ago. These painful lesions respond very well to acupuncture when the client seeks treatment soon after the outbreak. After two treatments, Jake's shingles had cleared up. Several months later, Jake came to see me very soon after heart surgery. One of his concerns was tachycardia- a very rapid heart rate. I treated Jake with acupuncture and herbs, and along with the hoped for result of his heart rate moderating, he experienced a deep feeling of well-being during and after his treatments. Before long, Jake was coming to see me for emotional issues as much as for physical issues.

The Heart in Chinese medicine is not equivalent to the physical organ that pumps blood as the central hub of our circulatory system. Heiner Fruehauf describes the Chinese notion of the Heart as an "empty vessel" and "container of *shen*" or spirit. (Appendix B, p. 108) The Chinese see the Heart as the Emperor, the center of consciousness. The Heart "... in its healthy state is capable of containing the fire of spirit, including the emotions and their potentially troublesome ramifications". (Fruehauf Appendix B, p. 109) In western thought, we also think of the heart as related to our emotions. We speak of "heartfelt" wishes, and there are countless songs "from the heart". These songs are referring to our emotional heart, not merely the physical organ that pumps blood.

Over the years that I have treated Jake, he told me about how his employer treated him and how his wife treated him. I began to have some notions of how unrelenting stresses in his life were experienced as injuries to his Heart, and may have contributed to his physical heart disease (along with his diet and his family history). As I recall my experience of supporting Jake's healing over more than 12 years, I express my interpretations of what he was going through. I can't honestly assert that I know or understand everything that was going on for Jake. I am certain that he would agree with me that his journey was one worth taking, that he is grateful to have made that journey, and that Chinese medicine treatments played a significant role in a deeply healing result.

Jake's warmth and enthusiasm come across immediately upon meeting him. He displays his interest in and appreciation of others readily. He loves to connect, laughs easily, and expresses his emotions directly, with feeling. A Five Element practitioner would likely conclude that he is displaying the Virtues of a healthy Fire element. How did a person like this find himself in a marriage to a manipulative, over-dramatic woman who could never be satisfied? And, how did Jake allow himself to continue to tolerate the angry outbursts, the unreasonable demands, and the absence of affection and respect? Jake is above all a "nice" person, coming from a Catholic upbringing. When he feels angry at how he's being treated, he does his best to understand the other person's perspective, and not to answer abuse with more abuse. Some psychotherapists might say that he turned his anger inward. Thea Elijah might see what she calls "angry doormat" syndrome. However he got into this situation, it was taking a toll on him.

When I asked to see Jake's tongue (to diagnose the state of his internal organs), I saw the results of years of emotional stress and frustration. When anger is not expressed over many years, the constraint of the heat of anger can show up in physical symptoms. All that heat can damage the *yin*- the calm, moist, cool, receptive principle that balances the *yang*- the hot, active, energetic principle within each of us.

Jake's pulse also showed how his vitality had been drained by those years of harsh treatment, and how even though he was drained, his body was on a sort of hyper-vigilant alert for the next onslaught.

Treating Jake with acupuncture, he often reported the positive effects of points being needled instantaneously as each needle is inserted. To treat Jake, I often choose points to nourish Jake's deficient *Yin*, calm his spirit, and smooth his constrained *qi*. Treatment with tuning forks after all the needles are inserted proves an effective way to deepen the effectiveness of Jake's acupuncture treatments. He invariably rests very deeply, often falling asleep during his time with needles.

As Jake came to recognize that his wife's lack of consideration for his feelings was a pattern not very likely to change, he found himself drawn to wearing woman's clothing and identifying himself as a "trans-gender" person. As he took steps toward divorcing his wife, he explored the possibility of sex-change surgery, and began spending time socializing with other 'trans' people in a neighboring community. After consulting with an endocrinologist, Jake began taking female hormones. I cautioned Jake to explore this direction slowly, with full medical supervision, to be sure that he wouldn't make a sudden change- for both his physical and emotional well-being. Recognizing that the divorce itself was a major change, I recommended that he give himself plenty of time to feel his way into his new life.

Jake bought and moved into a new home, got a couple of cats, and continued to have a relationship with his adopted daughter. His ex-wife demanded that Jake come to her home to make sure the daughter would be up and ready to go to school, and Jake found himself resenting these requests, while he went along with what his ex-wife asked him. In a class with Thea Elijah, I learned that a particular herbal formula could be helpful in maintaining appropriate boundaries. Since Jake's diagnostic signs fit the description of this formula, I prescribed it. The following week, Jake reported in a matter-of-fact way that he had decided to stop going to his former home to assume responsibilities that really belonged with his ex-wife. I smiled, silently thanking Thea and the Chinese herbs.

Another challenging situation for Jake arose at work, where he was accused of inappropriate sexual conduct toward other employees. Jake had "come out" to some of his co-workers, letting them know about his feelings about gender identity, and his exploration of a possible sex change operation, but he had never acted in a hurtful way toward anyone at work. Jake chose to contest the accusations, while making plans to finish his work at that agency and ultimately, he went to work on his own, contracting with several agencies. During this process which lasted several months, Jake received regular acupuncture, where he would tell me his updated situation, appreciate my supportive feedback, and then relax as acupuncture helped restore balance to his agitated spirit.

A couple of years ago, Jake began to date a woman whose husband had died a few years before. This relationship has been a source of great support and joy for Jake. While he still speaks as if he identifies as female, he's let me know that he's stopped looking into a sex change operation. He has also stopped socializing with his "trans" friends, who he'd never bonded with in a close way. After several major changes in his life, and exploring more dramatic changes, he seems very much at peace with his current life direction and his current relationship.

It's possible that some other approach to counseling might have put a stronger focus on Jake's interest in sex change, and may have identified it as a pathological rejection of himself. My experience working with Jake was my first time to counsel a person considering this sort of change (although I've known a few people who have gone through operations, who seem well-adjusted to their choice). When I consider the frustrating and lonely nature of the marriage Jake tolerated for years, I believe that he felt stuck in a situation which was lacking the possibility of deep connection, growth, or any healthy warmth and tenderness. The fact that Jake chose to explore his gender identity, while an unusual choice, may be looked at as a healthy way to consider some way to change from a situation that was unhealthy. If he felt totally frustrated as a male, there's a certain logic to considering what his life might be like as a woman. The Chinese usually consider movement and growth to be more healthy than stagnation. Jake moved away from stagnation, and he has grown. The fact that he now describes himself as deeply satisfied with his life, that he no longer feels the deep frustration and lack of satisfaction he experienced for many years, indicates that- regardless of how he feels about his gender- he has found a path to something that works for him.

If I were to speculate about what Jake's interest in sex change was about, I might tell myself a story that could explain Jake's experience in a way that might show off some psychological insights, and it would probably not be accurate.

Whatever I might imagine was going on is less important than the result: Jake left a marriage that had been emotionally harmful, established a better life for himself, including a more satisfying intimate friendship. He made use of acupuncture and Chinese herbs to support his evolution. It may not matter at all what it meant; what matters is that he expresses gratitude and joy in his new life, and he thanks his acupuncturist for being present during the changes that brought him to where he is today.

5

When Acupuncture Is Not Enough

Healing from significant emotional problems might require a combination of excellent psychotherapy with an energetic form of bodywork such as acupuncture, and other support. In the best of circumstances, a client will want her psychotherapist and acupuncturist to be able to discuss the work they are doing, and to work together toward agreed upon healing goals. Sometimes, family members and/or friends will also provide support. Healing deep emotional trauma is difficult, and is more likely to succeed with a good combination of supportive professionals working together.

Many people with serious emotional problems lack financial resources to pay for several different kinds of healers. Even when a person chooses to participate in psychotherapy and regular acupuncture treatment, it's common for the practitioners not to communicate about how they can best complement one another in working with their shared client.

A few years ago, a middle-aged woman saw me twice weekly for about six months in an attempt to emerge from a deep anxious depression, with delusional thinking and some psychotic features. Nancy had successfully run her own business, taught classes in the community, and previously recovered from a serious depression. This time, her situation seemed complicated by her awareness of her father's terminal illness, her unresolved ambivalence about her relationship with her father, and with other members of her family of origin.

Nancy was receiving counseling from the county mental health clinic, and was paying me about half my customary fee for her acupuncture treatments. I spoke on the phone periodically with her partner, and other supportive friends, but did not consult with her therapist.

As weeks went by, Nancy's hopelessness deepened, and she held more rigidly to the belief that nothing could ever change or help her return to a healthy outlook. Nancy's sleep was troubled, interrupted, and inadequate. She stopped working, canceled classes she had planned to teach, and undermined her relationships with friends by repeatedly changing planned times to meet, as she openly expressed a negative self-judgment about her own character and behavior.

Acupuncture usually provided temporary relief of these symptoms, allowing Nancy to sleep better, and plan on more positive activities to help her recover from her tailspin. But, the negative thinking and the confusion persisted for weeks, which turned into months.

I consulted with an acupuncturist colleague who had known Nancy when she was doing well, and got suggestions about her treatment. But, just as treatments seemed to be making a significant difference, Nancy decided to stop seeing me, claiming that she didn't want to keep feeling the discomfort of treatment with needles. I had been investing significant time and care in Nancy's treatment, and I felt troubled by her decision, but I wasn't sure what I could do. When someone decides to discontinue treatment, I usually respect that decision.

In retrospect, I regret allowing Nancy to discontinue treatment without asking to meet with her and discuss what wasn't working for her and help her consider what might work. While I want to respect any individual's choice about the treatments he or she chooses, I was aware of the severity of Nancy's condition, and I might have asked her to consider what plan might be best for her healing and recovery. I could have offered to keep treating her without needles. I can certainly treat people using tuning forks, shi-atsu massage, *moxibustion*, and other techniques that make use of my knowledge of Chinese medicine, and how to help calm a troubled spirit and smooth constrained *Qi*. But Nancy's hopelessness and persistent negative talk had worn down everyone in her life, to the point that her partner, her friends, and I had each come to see this deeply depressed and dysfunctional person might be the person who Nancy was going to be from now on unless something within her could make a change that was currently just not happening. We may have known a joyous, creative and skilled Nancy, and we'd been able to imagine a Nancy recovered from her depression, but months of persistent stagnation and lack of progress had taken a toll on our ability to see the virtues on the other side of Nancy's pathology.

Nancy seemed determined to destroy her healthy self. It's possible that another acupuncturist could have been more effective in seeing and nourishing the health that must have remained present beneath Nancy's severe pathology. If I had been thinking more creatively, I might have insisted that I meet with her therapist, and find out if bringing together several of the people who care about Nancy might contribute to her healing, something like the Chinese practitioners in the Wang Fengyi tradition bring together the entire community to witness the healing experience. When a group can gather to support a person in crisis, and acknowledge that we all know what it's like to feel hopeless and alone, sometimes there is more space for discovering creative alternatives and for a person like Nancy to feel better able to allow the group's healing intentions to overcome the habitual negative thinking.

I write about my work with Nancy here to acknowledge that there are times when treatment with acupuncture may not be enough to heal a serious emotional imbalance. While acupuncture seemed to play a useful role for Nancy, not enough other factors were firmly in place for the acupuncture to transform the pathological process , and the unhealthy part of her chose to discontinue the regular treatments and contact with me. The next time I am presented with a person in a comparably serious situation, I will attempt to collaborate with other practitioners, family members, and/or the client's support system to persist in seeking the necessary support and treatment for the person who is descending into madness. Persistence and creative thinking may be necessary when a seriously deep depression with psychotic features becomes a person's habit over a long period of time. There are situations where psychotropic medication and hospitalization may be the best available option to interrupt a deep pathological pattern, and only after some months of stabilizing from treatment with western medicine will a person like this be able to experience genuine emotional healing with Chinese medicine.

6

THE HEALING POWER OF CREATIVE EXPRESSION

When I was learning Shiatsu massage from Jim Cleaver in San Rafael, California in 1982-83, Jim spoke about the many aspects of living that the Chinese believe contribute to a balanced life. I remember Jim mentioning the person's family life, work life, the food he or she eats, martial arts practice, massage, creative expression (calligraphy, painting, or playing a musical instrument), Chinese herbal medicine, and if a person still wasn't living a healthy, balanced life after paying attention to all those things, acupuncture. I felt delighted to learn that the ancient Chinese believed that playing an instrument or doing calligraphy or painting was considered a healing and balancing pursuit. This wasn't the first time I'd heard this idea.

The first job I had after graduating from Cornell in 1972 was at the Austen Riggs Center, a private psychiatric hospital in Stockbridge, Massachusetts, which encouraged creative expression. My job description told me to be "available" to the patients in common areas. There were several chairs near the bottom of the staircase in the Inn where the residents lived, and that's where I'd often sit with whoever was wanting to be sociable. Occasionally, one of them would ask me to come with them on a walk outdoors, or to play a game of chess in the living room, or to talk. This hospital was not a locked facility. The young adults living there and seeing their therapists five days a week were free to walk down the road and spend time doing whatever they chose. Many of them chose to spend time making art in the Shop with the lavender door.

Joan Erikson, an artist and dancer (and wife of Erik Erikson, who was on the clinical staff at that time), began the Activities program at Riggs. These activities included doing all sorts of crafts and artwork such as throwing clay pots on the wheel in the Shop that was just three blocks from the Inn- where the people identified as "patients" resided. The Shop had a storefront, where crafts and artwork were sold, a large workspace, and upstairs a stage with seating for theater productions. Patients put on Ibsen's *Hedda Gabler* while I was working there.

My first week working at Riggs, I was encouraged to spend several hours doing the kinds of artistic things at the Shop that the patients were doing. I worked free form with clay (I sculpted the faces of two very old people- a man with a beard, and a woman wearing a bonnet); I painted with water colors (I remember a self portrait); and I don't recall what else I created there. But, I loved having the opportunity to do things I usually didn't do, and what I made spoke to me.

Many of the people residing at Austen Riggs were diagnosed with serious emotional problems, and a high percentage of them would line up at the nurse's station for medications in the evening and after breakfast. But, some of the residents didn't take any medications, and the philosophy of Riggs was that patients would participate in intensive psychotherapy, be given the lowest amount of drugs possible for them to be 'safe', and be free to express themselves artistically every day. At Riggs, the residents' inner experience came out into the community through the arts.

Michael Broffman, who speaks and writes Chinese with fluency, and practices his healing arts with great awareness of the Chinese traditions of healing, always encouraged my artistic expression (and the artistic expression of many of his clients). In 1987, Michael produced *The Ballad of 'Doc' Hay*, a play with songs, focusing on the first Chinese doctor to come to eastern Oregon in the late 19th century. Michael chose the playwright (Cherylene Lee), the director (Joya Cory), the songwriter (John Buckley), and I was invited to play mandolin as part of the small back-up group to support John as he performed his songs. The play was presented at the Marin Community Playhouse in San Anselmo, California, and at the Chinese Cultural Center in San Francisco's Chinatown. Every detail of the play's production was attended to by one of Michael's clients, fellow- healers and friends. This joyous project catalyzed new friendships, a strong sense of community, and other creative projects. From conversations with Michael, I came to recognize that he saw satisfying artistic expression serving a healing function.

When we look at Chinese writing, the characters are different from the English language letters you see on these pages: Chinese characters are symbolic representations of the ideas being conveyed. Stephen Cowan speaks of the healing power of symbols, as he speaks of the healing power of creativity. Birds building a nest are creating a safe place to nurture new life. A person using a brush to paint something is creating something new, something alive in the moment of its creation, something that touches other people and can catalyze feelings of recognition and self-recognition.

I've known many people who have made good use of creative expression to help heal traumatic experiences. One woman (an insightful and caring professional in her mid-50's) has two very troubled children. The older son became increasingly abusive of his mother in his late teens. The younger daughter became a drug addict. Over the years of many challenges and heartaches, this woman began to paint and draw. Beautiful colors in abstract paintings, and remarkably accurate self-portraits and portraits of her children flowed from her hand. Focusing her attention on creating something deeply satisfying to herself and others became a way to help her heal from the disappointments and feelings of loss she had experienced.

Several people I've known have found drumming to be a form of musical expression that helped them through frustrating, difficult times. The nonverbal, absolutely physical nature of playing any sort of hand drum- where the goal is to provide the steady heartbeat (or whatever more complex rhythms or poly-rhythms that more accomplished drummers play)- allows the drummer a meditative focus and a physical release. Drumming provides a way to be in close connection with others without having to go into all the specifics of the story of "how it's going". It's a great gift to experience the joy, precision and power (as well as the physical release) of drumming at any phase of our lives, but especially when healing from a traumatic or very challenging experience.

I've always loved music. I began playing guitar when I was 16, and I picked up my father's mandolin soon after that. I made up songs as soon as I could play a few chords, and by the time I was living out west around other songwriters, I began to consider myself a songwriter, too. It was satisfying to me to make a song out of my dreams, my experiences, my feelings, or stories or poems that moved me- and then sing my songs for others. I imagine that many songwriters work with painful and troubling experiences by writing and singing songs that express strong feelings, and work at a satisfying resolution. A disturbing relationship breakup, feeling betrayed by a family member or a lover- singing about these experiences exercises lungs that could be damaged by grief that doesn't move. The Chinese see value in moving the *qi*, rather than allowing it to stagnate, so that grief, anger, or sudden shock are less physiologically damaging if they move through the person when expressed in song.

Attending professional school to study Chinese medicine in mid-life was not an easy path for me (or several of my other middle aged classmates) to choose when I began acupuncture school at the age of 44. Memorizing point locations, and the actions and effects of hundreds Chinese herbs and herbal formulas would sometimes make my head spin. My herb teacher, Lu Weidong, knew that I was a musician, and he suggested I write songs about the herbs. He said that many Chinese would write poems to help them remember their herbs. I chose familiar melodies (from old folk songs, popular songs of my youth and Broadway shows) to write parodies to help me recall herbs to tonify Kidney Yang and calm a troubled Spirit (to the tunes of "Home on the Range" and "Let it Be" by Lennon and Mc-Cartney.) I would sing the songs to myself when taking exams, and can still recall some of them more than a dozen years after graduating from the New England School of Acupuncture. When a client presents me with a symptom I haven't treated in a long time, I often smile as a melody by Jackson Browne or Carole King comes to mind- with ingredients to an herbal formula in place of the original familiar lyrics. For those of us who remember song lyrics, this approach to memorization of information makes studying easier, because rhythm and melody and the act of singing all ground the information in the body, making for ready recall.

The act of creation, with its focusing of attention on what is being produced (be it musical sound, physical pieces of artwork, theatrical or dance pieces, or the writing of fiction), is a grounding and satisfying process in itself. The person creating the song or painting or story or dance begins with whatever in their living experience moves him or her to create; and in the movement of creating, an inner harmony is being re-established. When the song or story or painting is complete, the feeling of satisfaction is felt in the body; so that creation is healing in itself. And, the healing can continue, as the painting or song or play can be shared with an audience- of whatever size. Artwork can be appreciated by others, who can relate to the artist in ways that lead to a genuine sense of connection. Artists may write or sing or sculpt something for a particular person, and find that thousands of other people appreciate and benefit from the song or story or sculpture. In this way, the healing power of the artwork continues to serve, both the artist and the audience.

7

TRANSFORMATION OF FEAR TO WISDOM:
HEALING AND EMPOWERMENT IN THE 21ST CENTURY

While some of us may be more constitutionally predisposed to fear than others, living with existential fears has become a widespread way of experiencing our world since the development of nuclear weapons. My generation grew up in the era of "air raid drills," in which all the young children in every elementary school in America learned to respond to the sound of a siren by filing out of our classrooms into the hallway, kneeling in front of a row of lockers, and ducking our heads, anticipating a nuclear explosion. The fact that the Russians never did launch an attack on the US didn't change the experience of fear that millions of children remember vividly. We were kneeling, helpless, awaiting our destruction. We were never told what might happen after the bombs hit, so we were left to imagine our world shattered, many of our friends and family dead, and nothing as it had been before the dreaded attack.

Terrifying scenarios persist in our modern culture. Young children saw images of airplanes crashing into tall buildings in New York, the buildings collapsing in smoke and flames. The story is told of a child who saw the same images of the September 11 attacks on the family TV set repeatedly, who thought that plane after plane was crashing into building after building- that this sort of destruction was normal, and happened over and over again.

As we grow up, we sometimes learn that our parents and teachers may not have given us the most accurate or helpful explanations of the threats we face. And, if we continue to learn about our world, we come to realize that people in many places continue to be victims of random violence, and that the industries that fuel our economy have poisoned the water and air of communities with toxic chemicals. Our daily transportation in automobiles or airplanes is based on combustion of fossil fuels which are already changing our climate in ways that are likely to lead to dramatic changes in our ability to live as we've been living (especially if we live at low elevation near ocean or gulf coastlines). In the context of living with many disturbing aspects of life in the 21st century, how can we maintain a connection to the deep wisdom that is needed to make effective choices in our own lives in the midst of this complex world?

There's a lot to be afraid of. So, when a person comes to me complaining of anxiety or panic attacks, I want to assess what is causing the symptoms. I will consider who the person is constitutionally, what they experienced in their early family life, and how they understand their place in the larger community and society. Depending on the person, the goals could include tonification of Kidney *Yin* and *Yang*, moving congealed Blood from trauma (where the person has gone numb and repressed memories of the traumatic experience), and recommending activities that might be new and challenging, but that are definitely achievable. If the person has deep fears about the larger world, encouraging actions that contribute in a positive way to address large and frightening problems can help the person develop a way to live with joy and strength, even in the face of their fears.

"The lower (class of) medicines....govern the treatment of illness ...The middle class of medicines govern the nourishment of one's nature ....The upper class of medicines..... govern the nourishment of destiny ..." *Shen Nong Ben Cao* (8)

If a person suffers from panic attacks, one immediate goal is to alleviate the symptoms, so that the person can function in society. A second goal is to strengthen the person's overall vitality and sense of confidence, so that the person need not live in fear of having panicky responses to challenges in life. And the deepest goal, the "upper class of medicines" as the *Shen Nong Ben Cao* would put it, is to empower the person to participate in his or her community and society, and to dare to dream that their contribution might be "part of the solution" to the terrifying and numbing aspects of living in these times.

There are an infinite number of unique ways an individual can make a meaningful contribution. The gifted healer can help a person to identify a new direction, activity, or path and to experience joy in choosing to pursue that direction. Deciding to take in a foster child might speak deeply to one person, while volunteering for a political campaign will call clearly to somebody else. An artist might create a piece that honors all victims of violence, and a shy person might feel compelled to speak out in public for the health and safety of his or her community.

What the practitioner of Chinese medicine is looking to find are ways to release the person from the constraints that have held her back from expressing her genuine, heartfelt truth. As the person overcomes his or her fears and finds satisfying modes of self-expression, he or she can discover a deep source of power and wisdom within- which corresponds to the constitutional virtue on the other side of Fear.

True wisdom includes an awareness of the limits of what one person might be able to accomplish alone, and the power of what groups of people can accomplish together, over time. Some of my clients are already activists, attending 2 or 3 meetings daily, taking action out of a kind of desperation about the problems of the world; these people might need to take more time for quiet reflection and nourishment of their spirits. An over-committed activist might need to cultivate a faith that other caring people are also working for the causes of justice, human rights, and peace so that the activist can do his or her part, and rest with the knowledge that life goes on, whether or not the current crucial task gets addressed successfully. Losing an important vote in Congress can be very disappointing; working for a better world requires a resilience to tolerate disappointments, learn from them, and find effective ways to persist.

The activist who lives out the lyrics to the song by Sweet Honey in the Rock: "We who believe in freedom cannot rest" will not be a healthy or effective activist. Picture the anxiety-ridden insomniac activist, awake in bed at 3 a.m., repeating the lines to that song, thinking of all the things that need to be done, and still the big problems may never be solved.

It's not easy to find ways to thrive in our complex and threatened world. My activist friends have the intellectual understanding that taking on too many stressful responsibilities can bring on physical symptoms (such as headaches, an outbreak of shingles, or painful neck and shoulder tension.) Habitual over-work and over-worry will not help to achieve their goals. But, having that understanding may not be sufficient to allow the activist to actually rest from the challenges, to be able to bring forth the energy and clarity necessary to take effective action. And so, these activists come to me for acupuncture treatments, which alleviate stress-related physical complaints, and allow for deep relaxation. The activist can walk out of my office after a treatment with a renewed sense of aliveness and ease at living in his or her own body. The most effective of treatments will bring a shift in attitude as well as a feeling of physical well-being. The people who take action from their natural desire to love and protect rather than from their fear of losing will tend to live out a healthy balance of thought, action, recreation, and rest which will best serve their health and the health of their communities.

Five Animal Frolics:
Qi Gong and Tai Chi as Gateways to Inhabiting Our Own Bodies

Soon after I was first treated with acupuncture to alleviate severe back pain from a car accident in the early 1980's, I began learning *tai chi chuan*, in a class that Ellen Serber taught at the Pt. Reyes Dance Palace. I remember the first time I saw this small woman with wavy hair striding around the large room, adjusting the stance of her students by gently but firmly pulling down on the pelvis. And yes, she did that to me, too. I enjoyed the names of some of the moves: Repulse the Monkey, Single Whip, White Crane Flying, Wave Hands Like Clouds. And, I enjoyed doing the movements. When I finally learned the entire set, I practiced at home every morning, and felt more present in my body. I loved the variety of ways I could move- graceful and slow, then powerful with a kick or a punch.

After practicing a *tai chi* set, we were taught to stand, weight 70% on one foot, our arms encircling, as if we were embracing a tree, focusing attention on the lower abdomen, or *tan tian*. Dropping a lifetime of judgment about what activities were worthwhile and what activities were a foolish waste of time, I stood, arms encircling, breathing calmly into my belly. There was a pleasure in allowing my *tai chi* practice to be absorbed as I stood like a tree, rooted to where I was, feeling the air enter my lungs, pause, and let go.

Michael Broffman had suggested I practice *tai chi* to strengthen my back and lower body. I practiced every morning, first loosening up, then doing my kicks, and then moving through the form's slow dance until the routine was a steady part of my life. I would begin my day in a more calm and centered way. No matter what intense emotional things were going on in my life- news of serious illness of loved ones, conflicts with a family member, or the serious depression I went through while my mother and best friend were dying- I would wake up, loosen up, and do my *tai chi*.

Over the years, I have studied *tai chi* and *qi gong* with many gifted teachers: Rene Navarro, Paul Gallagher, my acupuncture school classmate Greg Dilisio, Fan Xiulan, and Josie Zhuo. While *tai chi chuan* is a martial art, with kicks and punches based on fighting, *qi gong* is a self-healing way of working with one's internal energies by moving and breathing, often imitating the natural world, in ways that will benefit every internal organ of the body. Each sequence, or set, provides movements that strengthen or stretch or otherwise enliven particular organs and energies of the body. Eventually, when some of my clients and friends asked me to teach a class in *Qi Gong*, it seemed natural for me to say, "Of course. Let me find a place and time".

Along with the pleasure of exposing other people to the benefits of *Qi Gong* practice, one of the great benefits to me was making the commitment to practice for a full hour with my students every time my class met. I always find it beneficial to do some *qi gong* and *tai chi* in the morning for 25 minutes or so. The experience of vibrant, glowing aliveness that comes after a full hour of *qi gong* was an extra bonus to teaching *qi gong* regularly.

When I spoke with the Ithaca Therapists Group about the value of acupuncture as an adjunctive treatment supportive of psychotherapy, I taught them "Five Animal Frolics" *qi gong*: the Crane, the Bear, the Monkey, the Deer, and the Tiger. Witnessing members of our psychotherapy community pouncing like a tiger going after her prey was a treat. My purpose in teaching these movements went beyond giving these people who spend too much time sitting in their offices the opportunity to move and have fun. Allowing a person who is anxious or depressed to attempt to embody the spirit of different animals allows that person to leave their mood behind as they imagine what it's like to soar in the air like a bird, crouch with the power of a bear, playfully tease like a monkey, establish watchful boundaries like a deer, or unleash the naked power of the predatory tiger. We all have a wider repertoire of actions and ways of being than we typically exhibit. Using the ancient Chinese *Qi Gong* forms to imitate the energies of wild animals allows all of us to move with greater expression and freedom, and to get unstuck from our habitual ways of moving, or not moving.

Among those of us who consider ourselves relatively healthy emotionally, a large number of us might admit that our lives can sometimes become unbalanced. Most of us work too much (or not enough), sit too much (or don't have the time to sit down), and spend too much time thinking seriously about all the things that seem too darn serious. Any practice of meditative movement provides an experience of awareness of the body and breath, and *Qi Gong* practices are designed to be easy to do so that the benefits are readily available to anyone who gives this approach a try. *Qi Gong* can provide a very easy way for any person to do self-healing. The ability to work with our own *qi* supports our self-esteem. It's true that email I read last night upset me. And, rather than responding immediately with an angry reaction, or staying awake for hours thinking over what was wrong with the person who wrote me such an annoying message, I can practice a Taoist *qi gong* exercise that Heiner Fruehauf taught at the Building Bridges Conference, shaking out all the tensions in the body, allowing the frozen areas to soften and melt away. I can breathe calmly, feeling the aliveness in my body. I can rest and sleep deeply, and find a more productive way to respond (or ignore) the provocative message that got me upset for a moment. We all can enjoy developing skills of self-care that we can practice anywhere we are, every day.

Although I had been aware of 'medical *Qi Gong*' for years, I first came to practice the *Zhi Neng Qi Gong* form after I happened to meet the Mexican artist Armando Santa Ana at a gallery exhibit of his work. Enjoying speaking in Spanish with the artist, I responded immediately to his offer to teach me a form I could teach my clients who suffered from serious illnesses. Both Armando's schedule and my schedule were more open than usual the week before Christmas in 2011. I agreed to meet him at 9am every morning for six days, practicing the routine of *Zhi Neng*, which includes visualization of sending golden light to enliven our cells and internal organs, imagining we can 'erase' negative emotions, and that we can affirm our lives and our close relationships as we move our hands like the crane. For me, learning in Spanish helped me receive the instructions without critical inner commentary, and I found that I was able to experience the benefits of the practice immediately, and with growing depth, as I continued to practice.

Soon after I completed this training with Armando, I introduced *Zhi Neng* to my *Qi Gong* classes. The response was so positive that I began setting up *Zhi Neng* workshops in other nearby cities, because I knew of nobody else teaching this form, and I felt moved to share the benefits with people in other communities.

In a way, the directions for the *Zhi Neng* form are like a form of hypnosis (or when one is practicing alone- self-hypnosis). A gifted hypnotherapist might suggest a healthier direction to his or her patients, and a teacher of *Zhi Neng* is suggesting that we can catalyze production of new red blood cells, and improve organ function by imagining we are sending the energy of golden light to our internal organs. Twenty years ago, I might have judged this entire pursuit as unscientific, and a waste of time. Today, it's hard to imagine a more productive use of one's time than to be using the powers of awareness and healing intention to nurture ourselves and our inner abilities to catalyze positive change.

9

Dream of the Red Chamber and Chinese Perspectives on Emotional Imbalance

Why do I find myself laughing, and feeling deeply satisfied, as I read a 17th century Chinese novel filled with mental instability, suicides, heartbreak, and disappointment? With characters constantly attempting to hide disturbing information from loved ones to protect them from being upset, allowing bad situations to get worse, I can see parallels to modern American families in a tale of 17th century China. When a gifted novelist portrays human nature as expressed in a particular culture with insight, the reader comes to know characters who- being true to themselves- make unhealthy choices, and suffer terrible consequences. As a reader, as it is with the reading of great works by Dickens, Tolstoy, and Cervantes, I nod my head and smile at the way the tale- outrageous and extreme as it may be- rings true.

Dream of the Red Chamber (also known as *The Story of the Stone*) by Tsao Hsueh-Chin brings the reader into the world of a wealthy Chinese family during its time of decline. But before the reader is introduced to Pao Yu, the "strange and unnatural" heir of the family, two immortals (a Buddhist monk and a Taoist priest) have a discussion with a jade stone with "supernatural powers" that is longing to travel in the "Red Dust" (or mortal life). The Stone, having served the Goddess of Disillusionment by caring for a Crimson Flower fairy plant- which has the habit to "feed upon the Fruit of Unfulfilled Love, and drink from the Fountain of Ineffable Sadness," is granted its wish, and is discovered in the mouth of the infant Pao Yu at his birth.

Pao Yu, described as "one of those exceptional beings who are born under a special set of circumstances and who are ...often misunderstood", wears the Stone on a cord surrounding his neck. Pao Yu's grandmother is the Matriarch presiding over the Chia family mansion called the Yungkuofu. The Matriarch takes special delight in Pao Yu, and also in his cousin, the sickly and unstable beauty Black Jade, who comes to live in the Yungkuofu with Pao Yu's sisters, and their numerous maids. Pao Yu delights in the company of all the girls, but feels a particular attachment to Black Jade from the moment of meeting her.

Soon after Black Jade moves to the Yungkuofu, Precious Virtue, another young girl who "showed a tact and understanding far beyond her years" arrives with her parents to take her place in the mansion, and "in a short time, Precious Virtue won the hearts of all..." She was "always ready to please and enter into the spirit of the occasion", whereas Black Jade "was inclined to haughtiness and held herself aloof".

As time passes, and Pao Yu (continuing to avoid the studies his father periodically admonishes him to get focused on so that he can do well on his exams) comes closer to the age of marrying, his grandmother and other relatives agree with Phoenix (Pao Yu's cousin who is in charge of running the household) that a marriage to Precious Virtue will be best for the young man's future, despite his deep and dramatic attachment to Black Jade. This marriage is seen as predestined, but because it counters Pao Yu's heartfelt love for Black Jade, it leaves Pao Yu confused and ill, while Black Jade dies after realizing that she has lost Pao Yu. Pao Yu's entire family conspires to deceive him about who he is marrying to the moment of the ceremony itself- when his dear Black Jade is nearing her death in her room, and Pao Yu is stunned to discover that Precious Virtue is his bride. For weeks after the marriage, the truth of Black Jade's death is kept secret from Pao Yu, as if he were still a child, unable to face the realities of life.

What does the reader find satisfying in a novel where many of the main characters and minor characters make ridiculously ineffective choices with tragic consequences as a result of their emotionally unstable characters? For example, we understand that San-chieh has a willful and dramatic nature. Liu Hsiang-lien (her potential suitor who has yet to meet her) initially sends his sword (which "has been in my family for generations and I have never parted with it" as a token of his commitment to San-chieh. However, Hsiang-lien reconsiders after asking Pao-yu about San-chieh and her family. He decides to break the engagement, and asks for the sword to be returned. In his first meeting with San-chieh, "as Hsiang-lien extended his hand to receive it, she pressed the keen edge of the sword to her throat... When they had recovered from the shock, San-chieh had already fallen dead." (p. 250) Hsiang-lien, in despair at losing "such a wife" cuts off his hair, and follows a Taoist priest 'we know not where'.

In our lives, we meet over-dramatic people, or may have over-dramatic tendencies ourselves. Fictional suicides like that of San-chieh, and the bizarre wedding of Pao Yu- in which he is misled about who he is marrying- are exaggerated situations that elicit powerful emotional reactions from the reader- a mixture of horror and outraged amusement.

Heiner Fruehauf tells of healers in northern China today who heal using the story-telling methods of Wang Feng-yi. People come with serious illnesses, listen to the healer tell stories which bring up powerful emotions, leading to cathartic laughter, crying, and vomiting. Pent-up toxic emotions are released, allowing for a deep feeling of relief, and what is described as genuine healing from serious illnesses such as diabetes and cancer. (Appendix B, p. 119)

It is possible that the lasting success of *Dream of the Red Chamber* comes from the strong feelings that the story brings up in the reader, who experiences shock, grief, and frustration at the tragic consequences of the emotional weaknesses of the characters. Because the extremes of the behavior and their consequences are outrageous and ridiculous, the reader might be moved to laugh, and to see the humor in the frustrating and ineffective behavior in their own family life.

Many minor characters enter the story, act our their sad and foolish vices, and quickly experience a sad downfall. For instance, Chia Jui, the lustful womanizer, pursues the competent and clever Phoenix. Arranging a late night rendezvous that she has no intention of attending, Phoenix sets up Chia Jui to be exposed to illness by waiting for her all night in the cold. When he finally receives the "Precious Mirror for Breeze and Moonlight" from the Goddess of Disillusionment, which is said to cure diseases resulting from impure thoughts and self destructive habits, Chia Jui does not follow the instructions to look only at one side of the mirror (which reflects a gruesome skeleton.) Instead, he looks at the forbidden side, which shows the woman of his dreams beckoning to him. Entranced and unable to resist, Chia Jui continues to look at the forbidden side of the mirror, exhausts himself with pleasure, and quickly dies.

The details of the ailments of the characters are central to *Dream of the Red Chamber.* In Chapter Six ("In Which Precious Virtue describes a Complicated Prescription"), she describes how to fill the prescription that gives her relief from feeling weak and short of breath:

"The ingredients...take time to assemble...you have to gather twelve ounces of white peony flowers which bloom in the spring, twelve ounces of white lotus flowers which bloom in the summer, twelve ounces of white lilies which bloom in the fall, and twelve ounces of plum flowers which bloom in the winter. These flowers must be dried and ground up on the following vernal equinox and mixed with the powder that the monk left with us. For this purpose one must have twelve *ch'ien* of rain water that falls on the day of Rain Begins-" Other characters express outrage at the ridiculously time-consuming process, but Precious Virtue takes it in stride. "...By a series of happy coincidences, we got everything in about two years and made a supply of the pills."

Even more central to the novel is the notion that emotions contribute to, or even cause, illness.

Pao Yu says to Black Jade: "You are now burdened with illness largely because you worry too much..." (p. 160)

Attempts are made to treat the pathological conditions of Pao Yu and Black Jade, but all these interventions fail in achieving genuine emotional healing. Doctors are called in, they prescribe herbs, but the conditions are found to be too extreme and persistent in these characters to make a lasting difference.

The main strategy chosen to avoid the negative consequences of Pao Yu becoming extremely upset (and exhibiting the agitation and wild behavior associated with his upsets) is to withhold information that might be upsetting, trying to keep him as calm as possible. The underlying assumption seems to be that life presents situations that are going to be overwhelming and intolerable to a weak personality type with a delicate constitution, so the only answer is to protect this sort of person from awareness of what life brings. Because Pao Yu is treated as a privileged child, expected to say and do extreme things, nobody in his world demands that he behave more responsibly. His father's angry reminders to study for his exams seem to be experienced as an unpleasant storm rather than any sort of guidance toward living a responsible life.

In the novel, there are no truly gifted healers to help Pao Yu or Black Jade. There is no hands-on intervention- no acupuncture or massage- to provide a transforming experience of balance and peace. No teacher provides grounding practices of *Qi Gong* or meditation, and nobody gives insightful guidance about how Pao Yu or Black Jade might learn to cope and live with the challenges of their unique constitutional natures.

Pao Yu is a child who never matures. His father Chia Cheng is mostly absent, and the father's visits with Pao Yu are not seen as supportive. Chia Cheng repeatedly admonishes Pao Yu to study for his examinations, but he never shows any fondness, appreciation or interest in Pao Yu's feelings. Pao Yu grows up without the experience of witnessing an adult male taking a healthy place in family interactions. And, because Pao Yu never leaves the Yungkuofu, never goes out to school, he never has to face the challenges of dealing with any other people, and never has to negotiate cooperative working relationships. He never encounters a male role model who embodies the virtues of moderation and caring participation in family life that could show him a way he might eventually succeed in the world.

Black Jade's family sent her to live with her cousins, perhaps because they would prefer not having to deal with a demanding, narcissistic complainer. Nobody in the Yung-kuofu confronts Black Jade's off-putting actions; rather, they avoid her. Her beauty is somehow seen as an excuse for her immaturity. She is always seen as fragile, constantly on the verge of illness, and medicines do very little to help her transcend this fragility.

The jade stone deemed to have supernatural healing powers offers Pao Yu his only protection from insanity; when it is lost, Pao Yu becomes totally incapable of coping successfully with emotional challenges. He is left with no will to act in a way that can satisfy his Heart's desire.

The deeper message of the story may be that when Pao Yu accommodates to the conventional choices foisted upon him by his elders (and allows himself to be separated from Black Jade), he falls into confusion and illness. Had Pao Yu had the strength to resist the manipulations of Phoenix and the household, he might have honored his own Heart and true nature, and found a way to health (and a lasting relationship with his beloved Black Jade).

Because this novel's story tells of "unfulfilled love" and 'ineffable sadness," Pao Yu's weakness and confusion are no match for the manipulations of Phoenix, and the tragic loss of Black Jade is the result. With the Buddhist monk and the Taoist priest asserting that mortal life is inevitably suffering, we are asked to accept that people will continue to remain stuck in dysfunctional patterns rather than rising to the challenge to learn and grow emotionally so as to overcome their challenges.

The dream referred to in the title of the novel is the one source of insight that comes to Pao Yu. The goddess who comes to Pao Yu in the dream to tell him what his personality is like provides him with an experience of intimacy with a woman with characteristics of both Black Jade and Precious Virtue.

Understanding this dream could have helped prepare him for relationships with the women in his life. Unfortunately, the dream seems to be forgotten later in the story, and Pao Yu's descent into a disconnected and ineffectual state prevents him from taking any actions to avoid tragedy.

None of us wants to suffer the tragic fate of Black Jade and Pao Yu, or see our friends, family, or clients suffer similar fates. As practitioners of psychotherapy or Chinese medicine, we don't want to merely offer an herbal formula or a pharmaceutical to allow clients with immature and dysfunctional personalities to "cope" or survive. Certainly, we want to alleviate uncomfortable symptoms, and we also want to help catalyze healthy maturation so that our clients become the selves they've always felt they might become. Had Pao Yu found a truly effective healer, the novel would not have retained its tragic power.

Pao Yu is merely a cautionary fictional character. Many young adults who have led sheltered lives may have some qualities in common with Pao Yu. As practitioners of healing arts, it's our job to find ways to catalyze growth, and not to enable families to keep young people sheltered from opportunities to grow into whole adult human beings. Many young people experience psychotic breakdowns in their teens and early twenties. The easy accessibility of mind-altering drugs may have increased the frequency of these experiences in the past few decades. A mental health system that assumes that a person who has suffered a breakdown needs to take anti-psychotic medication for the rest of their lives is a system that denies the possibility of genuine healing.

The transition from adolescence to young adulthood can be tumultuous for many young people. Changing bodies, changing hormones and multiple options of social roles regarding intimacy, sexuality, and life direction can lead to powerful feelings and the possibility of being overwhelmed. Going through a crisis is no reason to relegate a young person to the role of mental patient. Healers who are trained to look for the virtues underlying the pathologies they see in their clients are more likely to support young people to find their way past breakdowns in ways that give them freedom and choices. A skilled practitioner might insist that a young person take on responsibilities suited to his or her growing capabilities. The work of healers includes helping our clients grow in their abilities to work effectively with their emotional responses to life's challenges, so that they might avoid the dire consequences described in novels like *Dream of the Red Chamber*.

10

CHINESE MEDICINE AND THE END OF LIFE

When I decided to study Chinese medicine, I didn't realize how important a role acupuncture could play for people at the end of their lives. Most of us have witnessed people suffering in their last weeks. Acupuncture treatments may not be able to cure cancer, but I've seen acupuncture help make people far more comfortable in their final weeks of life. Each person I've treated in their last days seems to have benefited in ways beyond just being more comfortable. Each, in their own way, has been better able to maintain their abilities to interact as they wanted, and as a result, come to more satisfying completions of their closest relationships.

When I was a child growing up, my family shared Thanksgivings and other major occasions with a family in the neighborhood who had three children about the same ages as my siblings and me. Debbie was my age, and she was the first person I treated with acupuncture in the last week of her life. Debbie had been living in Harrisburg, PA in 1978, when the accident at the Three Mile Island nuclear power plant released radiation that may have contributed to the cancers that showed up in her body 15 years later.

The summer after I graduated from acupuncture school, Debbie was at her parents' home, weak and dizzy from the cancer that had metastasized to her brain. She found the dizziness intolerable, because it so dominated her awareness. When she heard I might be coming to visit, she asked me to treat her with acupuncture. Newly licensed and just opening my practice, I called Michael Broffman for advice about how I might treat Debbie, never having treated someone in such a frail condition. Michael asked me questions about what I thought was causing the dizziness, and helped me come up with a plan of points to needle. Once the needles were inserted, Debbie said, "Soft." She rested for about 15 minutes, then turned to me, and asked how I'd been doing. She seemed so happy to be able to have an ordinary visit with an old friend. I treated Debbie for three days in a row, and she was able to feel calm and at ease. When I said goodbye to her, she asked me in a matter-of-fact way to call her next time I was in town; two days later, I learned that she had died.

I've had similar experiences treating other people who were nearing death; the acupuncture would alleviate symptoms: pain, coughing, dizziness, nausea . Once the uncomfortable symptoms eased off, the person would relax and enjoy talking with me. One client's sister called to let me know when her sister had passed away, and she told me that my client had said that the times having acupuncture with me were the most peaceful and comfortable times of her last several months.

Most Americans who receive a cancer diagnosis choose to have western medical treatments- surgery, chemotherapy, and/or radiation. A typical role of Chinese medicine in these situations is helping to make the person more comfortable, and to boost vitality and digestive functioning in the context of the harsh western treatments. Research done by the Pine Street Foundation has found that integrating traditional Chinese Medicine with Chemotherapy can enhance the likelihood of survival for several forms of cancer, and I've used herbal protocols from Michael Broffman to support a good friend who is now thriving after her bout with cancer. (Michael Broffman, L.Ac. and Michael Mc-Culloch, MPH, L.Ac.,"Integrative Traditional Chinese Medicine and Chemotherapy: Survival Data in Node-Positive and Metastatic Breast Cancer" in *San Francisco Medicine: Journal of the San Francisco Medical Society*, November-December, 2001)

Rarely, a person who receives a cancer diagnosis chooses not to receive Western treatments, based on a judgment that these treatments are unlikely to extend the length of life very much, and are very likely to have a negative impact on quality of life. James, a 74 year old man who had been on dialysis for five years and carried around an oxygen tank to help him breathe, decided that chemotherapy for his bladder cancer was likely to increase his discomfort. He chose treatment with acupuncture and herbs to support his vitality and alleviate various symptoms that came up in his final phase of life. I encouraged James to consult regularly with his oncologist, and consider the western medical recommendations; James was interested to receive diagnostic information from his doctors, but he rejected all recommended Western treatment options.

As James' condition deteriorated over time, he would celebrate any return of normal functioning. After several weeks of nausea, zero appetite and very low energy, his acupuncture treatments enabled him to take deep pleasure in eating when his appetite returned, and increased his ability to be more physically active. James wanted more physical movement, so he attended several *Qi Gong* classes I was leading. I can recall his delight at doing the Five Animal Frolics Qi Gong, allowing himself to enter the spirit of each animal as he soared gracefully like a crane in flight, and pounced fiercely, like a tiger leaping upon its prey. A week after our last *Qi Gong* class, James asked me to come treat him in his apartment because he didn't feel safe driving himself the few blocks to my office. Once he was resting comfortably with needles, he directed me to read a short story he'd had published in a literary magazine a few decades ago. He was aware that his time was getting short, and now that I was in his home space, he wanted to share more of himself, and of who he'd been when he was younger, and more vital.

The following week, James called to cancel his acupuncture appointment, saying he could barely stand up. He asked me to come treat him at the Hospice residence where he'd be going. He had decided to discontinue dialysis, which he was finding increasingly uncomfortable, and in that decision, he was choosing to die.

The morning I visited James at the Hospice, he was sitting with his daughter-in-law, enjoying his breakfast, marveling at the changes he was going through. He said to us, "I don't know if I'm going through a breakdown or a breakthrough. The past 24 hours has been so amazing, I'd like to write a novel about it." The phone rang: it was his son, who had driven 500 miles to see him. James told him: "My acupuncturist is here. He's helping me". I wasn't sure what he meant, but his spirits seemed light and warm.

After he finished eating, James wanted to get up and go for a walk, but first he wanted to use the bathroom. He called a nurse to help him, and while in the bathroom, he lost consciousness. The nurse called for help. I joined her in holding James up, asking James if he could hear me, noticing him gasp for a few breaths, and then stop breathing. The nurse asked me to run for another nurse. I ran off, and when we returned, James was gone.

Both James' sons arrived within a half hour, and I later joined them for the burial and memorial service. Being present with James during his last hour alive felt like a blessing to me, especially to witness his courage and openness and curiosity about the process of dying. I can't know with certainty about James' experience of acupuncture during his last year alive, beyond knowing that he came regularly, he said he would have wanted to come more often, if he hadn't needed to be on dialysis 3 days a week, and that he'd come to feel that the presence of his acupuncturist was somehow helping him as he faced his dying.

Most of us consider an anxious preoccupation with what might go wrong in the future to be characteristic of a neurotic personality (exemplified in the characters portrayed by Woody Allen in his many movies). A healthy attitude toward the future is one in which the person prepares for and plans for changes that are coming with some combination of anxiety, curiosity, and wonder. Dying may be the most profound change in our future, and I believe it's valid to consider whether our attitude toward our own death is relatively healthy or perhaps unhealthy.

Thea Elijah teaches what she calls a 'Perennial Medicine' approach to Chinese Medicine. Thea says:

"The most significant aspect of any system of medicine is not the technicalities of how the healing is implemented, but whether that system of medicine orients itself in relation to a central model of perfection, which constitutes both the goal and the agency of healing, or whether it orients itself in relation to the dispelling of illness and the avoidance of death." Thea is talking about a universal goal found in all religious traditions, including traditions that do not recognize a Supreme Being : to seek an experience of unity with all-that-is, however that may be described or named. Where Christians and Jews speak of God, Muslims speak of Allah, the Chinese may say the Tao, or the Way. For people who do not feel any connection with a religious tradition, this experience may come as sense of connection

with Nature, or Humanity, or the Earth, or future generations.

Thea asserts, "the extent to which you achieve realization
of unity within your lifetime, you will be glad that you did
when you die. This is ....a whole orientation towards why
we live, and what is health, and what is it that we are actually aiming for. Just not to die for a little bit longer? Or to
make ready for what state we will be in when we die."

And, "when we focus solely on dispelling illness in order
to restore health a priceless opportunity for the spirit is lost.
When our healing strategy has as its aim the evocation of
the client's own original nature as its catalyst for the transformation of body, mind and spirit, the results are profound
for both practitioner and client. The client experiences
healing as a transformation that occurs from within; and
the practitioner is also transformed through the continuous
practice of aligning with The Most High in ourselves for
the sake of our client." (9)

I quote Thea at length because her words speak to what
happened to me during the many months I spent treating
James. I truly wanted to support James in feeling as genu-
inely alive as he could, despite his multiple physical challenges. By sharing as much of James' last months with him
as I did, I find myself changed. James did not appear to be
afraid as he faced his death; he was curious, and fascinated,
and wanting to share the experience with others.

I cried in the moments after James was gone, as his body
was growing cold. I had come to feel close to James during
the many months he came for treatment, and increasingly

so as he made choice after choice to live every moment he had with awareness and appreciation. The contrast between feeling James' alert and engaging presence one moment and then seeing the body that he had just left behind was profound to me, and my tears came from a genuine grief at the loss of my relationship with him. From talking cheerfully and enjoying his last meal, James got up and left us. He didn't appear to be suffering. He appeared to be at peace.

I'm grateful to all my teachers of healing in the East Asian traditions from China and Japan. There is something both miraculous and absolutely ordinary about the practice of Oriental Medicine. In life, we all can get out of balance. We suffer losses. We get sick. We make mistakes. The techniques I've learned from my teachers have helped alleviate pain and suffering, have helped people discover a way out of habitual misery, and have eased the transition out of this life into the mystery.

People ask me how acupuncture works. I smile and say one of these things: "Magic." "Moving the *qi*". Or, "I don't know." When I insert needles into a person's body, I know my intention is to catalyze a shift toward greater harmony and balance, but I honestly don't know for certain what will happen. Most of the time, something useful, gentle, and 'soft' as my old friend Debbie said, happens. And that something is frequently a movement toward healing.

Appendix A

Healing Emotions in Children

by Stephen Cowan, MD
2012

The Diagnostic Statistical Manual (DSM), the bible of conventional Western psychiatry, has been relatively effective in providing detailed categorization of what's *wrong* with us, but it doesn't really tell us what is *right* with us. This presents a significant problem when it comes to growing a healthy child in your house or your practice.

The explosive rise in the diagnosis of children with mental disorders over the past 20 years has led to significant overuse of strong psycho-pharmaceutical medications originally intended for adults and not FDA approved for pediatric use.[1] This has several untoward effects. It often puts clinicians in the difficult position of *having* to treat a child once a diagnosis has been given or run the risk of malpractice. A recent report in the Harvard Medical Letter has gone so far as to suggest that the wide availability of psycho-pharmaceuticals may actually be influencing the clinician's process of diagnosis. [2] DSM diagnoses are based on the collection of symptoms, not pathophysiology, and treatment options can give the false impression that each symptom has a distinct neurochemical association. Treating symptoms as if they are diseases promotes quick fix solutions that suppress natural physiologic processes and ignore the causes underlying those symptoms. Contrary to what pharmaceutical companies would like you to believe, the promise of "better living through chemistry" can leave us crippled by a life-long dependency on pills without ever probing the deeper roots of our emotional problems. In children, there are subtler problems in labeling emotional disorders.

The increase in diagnostic labeling of emotional disorders in children has led to a trend in over-identification with their diagnosis. It is not uncommon these days to hear kids say "I'm ADD" or "I'm bipolar" as if the label were somehow genetically written into their identity. When a child identifies herself with such artificial labels, it can contribute to a pervasive sense of psychological helplessness that prohibits full recovery. Furthermore, the use of "adult" psychiatric diagnostic criteria in children ignores the very qualities that define children as different from adults, namely their ever-changing process of growth and development. Children are not just "little adults." Many of their symptoms are transient responses to contextual challenges that promote adaptation and growth. There is little research to support the validity of correspondences between adult and child psychiatric diagnoses and a significant lack of long-term studies on the safety and efficacy of using adult psychiatric medications in children. The intensity and vibrancy of changing behaviors is what makes children so much fun to be around. Their wondrous sense of exploration and creativity makes each child much less predictable particularly when it comes to labeling and treating emotional states.

But perhaps the biggest problem concerning the DSM is the complete lack of any definition of "emotional health," which gives the impression that health is simply the absence of a diagnosis. But there is more to living a healthy emotional life than *not* having a label.

Resilience

The plasticity of a child's nervous system captures the concept of *epigenetics* that has revolutionized our understanding of the interrelationship between our hereditary and environmental influences. Rather than seeing ourselves from the perspective of hardwired genetic determinism, we now have a broader ecological view of what it means to be healthy. This is particularly important in defining emotional health in the growing child.

Mark Greenberg, the noted psychologist at Penn State University has done groundbreaking work in investigating the factors that determine how we cope with what Hans Selye called "the stress of life."[3] Stress is a necessary stimulus for growth and adaptation, and can be defined as how well we bend and recover from the winds of change. Our coping mechanisms are directly influenced by our circumstances and temperament. The more labels we place on children based on statistical analysis, the less tolerant we are towards children whose adaptive styles don't "fit" neatly into the rigid expectations of how a child should behave. The smaller the box, the more kids fall out of it. The less tolerant, the less likely we are to look at the environmental factors that may be contributing to a child's emotional distress. This is often a case of blaming the victim. The epidemic use of psychiatric medications in children has its roots in such narrow perspectives. The first step in understanding how to improve an individual child's emotional health is to widen our perspective, to look beyond the small view that reduces that child to genes and chemistry and take note of the diverse factors that support or interfere with his resilience.

The Mandala of Epigenetic Fitness

We are living communities rather than isolated individuals. An expanded view of who we are must first consider the fact that 99% of the proteins made in our body derive from non-human microbial cells living primarily in our gut. What's more, each bite of food we take contains genetic material that directly influences how our genes express themselves. The health of our gut community has a direct effect on our emotions. For example, over 80% of the mood-stabilizing hormone serotonin produced in the body is made in the gastrointestinal system. We communicate with the world through our gut and in reality our gut is like a brain that directly regulates our mood.

But to truly think outside the box, we must appreciate the total matrix within which a child lives. The burgeoning field of *behavioral epigenetics* championed by Moshe Szyf at Mcgill University is just beginning to give us a glimpse of how interconnected our emotions and behaviors are to the subtle environment around us.[4] In exploring factors that contribute to what I call "epigenetic fitness" we need to look at the mandala of our life (see diagram). *Mandala* is an ancient Sanskrit word that means relationship. How we relate and are related directly influences our epigenetic fitness. This is the key to promoting emotional wellbeing.

The Epigenetic Mandala

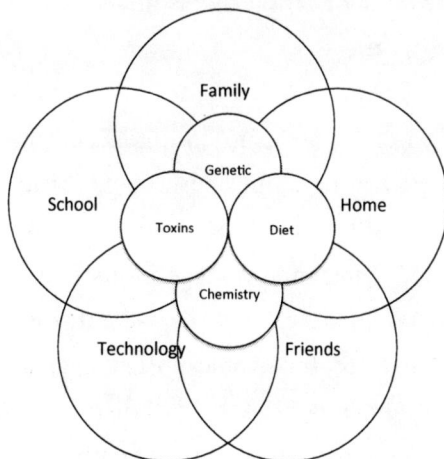

©Cowan 2012

Food: The quality of the food our children eat certainly affects their emotional stability. The current obesity epidemic is directly related to the rise in high-energy, nutrient-poor foods that alter blood sugar balances, shorten frustration thresholds and drive compulsive behaviors. But it's not just what we eat but where we eat, how we eat, when we eat and why we eat that determines our emotional well-being. The sensory experience of eating is one of the most primal ways we relate to the world. Hunger is a powerful motivator and distractor depending on our attitudes and habits of eating. Many children today over-indulge in mindless eating of poor quality fast food, leaving no time to properly process nutrients. This leads to accumulations that cause inflammation of the gut and phlegm that "mists the mind." More importantly they have lost the deeper meaning of eating that is linked to how we connect with others.

Toxins: We are exposed to toxic environmental factors every day. Our physical and emotional health is affected by cumulative burden of toxins that come from living in a modern industrialized world. The air we breathe, the food we eat, the noise we are exposed to, the over-exposure to artificial light, artificial heat and cooling all disrupt our connections with the natural rhythms of daily life. Lack of sleep and exercise trigger chronic stress hormone depletion resulting in endless bouts of physical pain and fatigue, cognitive exhaustion and erratic emotions. Because children are growing at such rapid rates, they are particularly prone to depletion. They are "the canaries in the coal mine."

Family: Our family serves as our primal support system. Family dynamics can also become as toxic as chemical exposures. Emotions are contagious and a child can be caught in an echo-chamber of emotional distress when her family is not supportive or stable. Mary Ainsworth, a pioneer in the field of child psychology attachment theory has described the importance of a secure base as essential for emotional health and resilience.[5]

Friends: How often does a clinician consider asking friends to participate in the treatment of a child with emotional disorders? There are many times in my career when a patient's friends have come forth with valuable information that helps illuminate what is really going on in my patient's life. This is particularly true with teenagers who have evolved their own supportive social network. The recent rise in online bullying has highlighted the dark side of such exposures and needs to be investigated carefully.

Home: The structure and setting of the house where a child lives can have powerful effects on her emotional state. Which side of the bed she sleeps on, the color of the walls, where she eats, where she plays will all contribute to the resilience of a child.

The ancient Chinese practice of *fengshui* looks at the subtle ways we can shift mood by altering the look of one's home to promote greater harmony and positive emotional states.

Technology: Perhaps the most underappreciated influence on our children's emotional resilience lies in their exposure to modern digital technology. Our children are considered "digital natives," having grown up fluently speaking the language of the internet, cell phones and videogames. We adults are "digital immigrants." We may be able to speak the language but it is not necessarily natural to us. Adapting to the highly visual, over-stimulating world of technology can leave children feeling isolated, bored and apathetic in environments like school where they do not have access to the same kind of feedback.

School: We must not forget the powerful effect our schools have on our children's emotional wellbeing. As our schools become more rigid in their standardized institutionalization of learning, there is less and less tolerance for the diverse ways children adapt, grow and express themselves. This is perhaps one of the most common causes for over-labeling children with psychiatric disorders.

A child resonates with each of these fields and they are

all interconnected. Each can be used therapeutically to enhance a child's ability to recover from emotional distress effectively without medication.

Tong: the true meaning of health

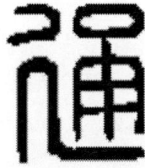

The classical Chinese symbol *Tong* shows the image of movement next to a bell ringing. It means to connect, to communicate, to open up, to clear. Free-flowing communication defines what it means to be healthy from a Chinese medicine perspective. How well a child resonates with the fields of his life will determine his emotional wellbeing. An emotional illness can be understood to be a communication breakdown within the epigenetic mandala. Building emotional resilience in children therefore begins by working with the power of resonance in order to promote what I call "emotional immunity."

There are many misconceptions about the meaning of immunity. As a holistic pediatrician I often explain to parents that a strong immune system does not mean one never gets sick. That would actually be very abnormal. It is how we recover that defines the power of the immune system. The immune system is an integral part of our consciousness. A healthy immune system has the capacity to listen and speak to the world. It has memory, vigilance and responsiveness but most importantly, it has the power to let go and returns to a state of listening. Emotional immunity does not mean never feeling upset. Its power lies in its flexibility and focus.

The Cycle of Emotional Recovery

I see my job as a holistic health care provider as promoting recovery in children, not simply putting out fires by treating symptoms. To promote emotional recovery we must take a closer look at the relationship between feelings, emotions and behaviors. (see diagram)

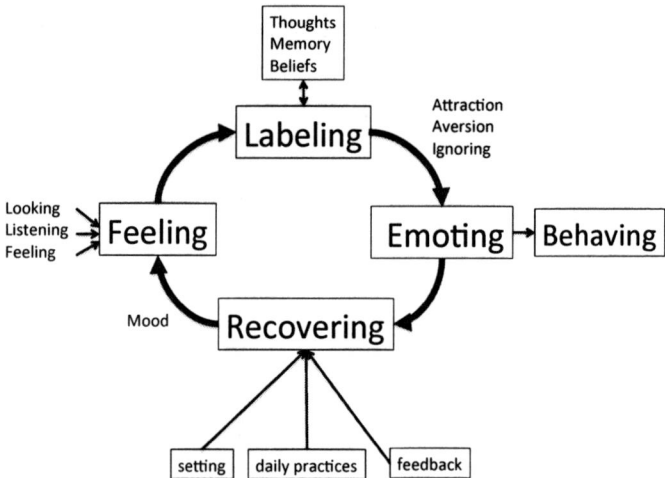

©Cowan 2012

Life is a delicate balance of movements. The primal doorway to resonating with the world lies in our sensory experience. Listening, looking, smelling, tasting and feeling are literally how we vibrate with the world. Within seconds, the open-ended experience of life begins to be labeled, categorized and conceptualized into good or bad or neutral. We begin to hear, see and touch *something*. As a child develops language, memory and beliefs shape sensory experience into a personal reference system. Neuroscience has demonstrated that there is a gap of about 200 milliseconds between sensation and the categorization of these feelings. As the sense of Self begins to solidify in early childhood, labeling helps internalize experience by refining the direction of primary sensory movements into specific attractions, aversions and ignoring. Each child has a unique style and direction that manifests in specific facial expressions, body language, tone of voice that Antonia Dimassio calls Emoting[6]. Expressions of this internal motion or "emotion" is how we dialogue with the world as we experience it. This is the evocative aspect of *tong*. How effectively we emote reflects the nature of our security at any given moment in the world.

Emotions in turn activate the movement of behaviors that serve to promote responses in the world. In a sense this is the other side of the tong-conversation. In young children, the speed with which feelings take shape as emotions and behaviors can be terrifying for them and daunting for parents. I often compare them to barking puppies. A child who is in a chronically insecure state may become so swept away by the sheer intensity of her emotions that she is unable to manifest what I call her "Big Heartedness." Big heartedness is a child's ability to sense the big picture of her life and communicate with her innate creativity, wisdom and compassion in the world. For the immature child, feelings become emotional impulses with such lightning speed that they can set up vicious cycles of emotional instability. Young children are not able to distinguish between feelings, emotions and behaviors. When told to stop a behavior, they will often think this means *stop feeling*. This can be a dangerous path to suppression of feelings and emotions that will manifest in deep-seated psychological pathologies later in life. As I explain to children, while there are certainly inappropriate behaviors, there are no inappropriate feelings.

If tong-communication is a key to emotional health, learning to effectively label feelings is an important way of building space to experience emotions as they arise without becoming overwhelmed. Most importantly, teaching children that their emotions do not define who they are is a central focus of my work. When children learn to notice how their emotions come and go, there is more space for recovery to take place. A recent long-term study that followed children for 30 years demonstrated that developing emotional regulation was a primary factor in ultimate outcomes of economic success, social success and physical health.[7]

Much of my work with parents and children lies not only in learning to notice how feelings become emotions but also in learning to notice how to let go of strong emotions and return to feeling. The recovery process is directly influenced by a child's setting, the feedback she receives and her personal daily practices (qigong breathing, meditation, visualizations, chanting, prayer, etc.). But one size does not fit all kids. When the setting does fit the nature of the child, he may be unable to let go of an emotion. Lingering moods will then distort the clarity of sensory experience, amplifying perceptions and setting up vicious cycles of confusion and distress that fuels chronic pathological behaviors. This can interfere with the natural dialogue necessary for learning, memory and a sense of wellbeing in the world.

Preparing children for emotional stress without instigating fear is a way of empowering them to recover effectively, rather than viewing symptoms of distress as failure. This is a revolutionary concept in health care. Shortening recovery time puts a different spin on how you live your life and interact with others. This changes the mood of healing and clarifies the goals of therapy. At each phase along the cycle of feeling-labeling-emoting-recovering, there are opportunities to empower a child to effectively express their emotions and with practice return to a state of emotional clarity of heart.

Xin: The Motion of Heart

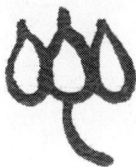

We are wired to pay attention. Every aspect of our nervous system is designed to resonate with the world. Attention allows us to connect to the world and integrate it into our being. As the eminent father of psychology, William James said, "That which I choose to pay attention to, shapes my brain." Learning how to pay careful attention to feelings as they arise creates an intimate connection with the cycle of emotional recovery.

In Chinese medicine, the idea of mind and heart are held within one term: *xin*. This ancient character shows what some believe to be a lotus blossom opening with a stem and three leaves. Others say it represents the chambers of the heart. There is deep meaning in this imagery. As a pediatric neurodevelopmental specialist, I find that something marvelous happens when we replace the word "mind" with "heart." Moving beyond a reductive model based in wiring and chemistry towards a more organic sense of how we open up to the world offers a radical perspective on what it means to pay attention with all our heart. In my book, *Fire Child Water Child*, I describe my approach to helping children develop their unique styles of attention and become masters of their Big Hearted emotions.[8]

In my practice I teach children how to become connoisseurs of their heart by using their power of imagination. By noticing the movement of feelings and developing symbolic language to describe them as they arise without judgment, children increase their awareness of the ways feelings shimmer and shift. This brings greater shades and colors to the emotional landscape. When children are given a chance to examine the subtle movements of their senses, they don't get swept away by emotions as they arise. As they gain greater confidence, they find it easier to let go of strong emotional states and clear the perceptual clouding that comes from residual moods. This is the foundation of emotional resilience.

The Motion of Emotion

The Chinese medical perspective offers a refreshing view of emotion. The motion of feelings and the emotions that emerge are a reflection of the movement of *Qi* within our experience of life. In the early Lingshu texts, each emotion has a characteristic movement, direction and purpose, corresponding to a seasonal phases (Spring-Wood, Summer-Fire, Harvest-Earth, Autumn-Metal, Winter-Water). These movements resonate in corresponding organ networks (liver, heart, spleen, lung, kidney) and have particular physical, cognitive and emotional patterns. I have developed a set of simple icons to help children and parents identify with these movements (see diagram).

The Movements of Qi

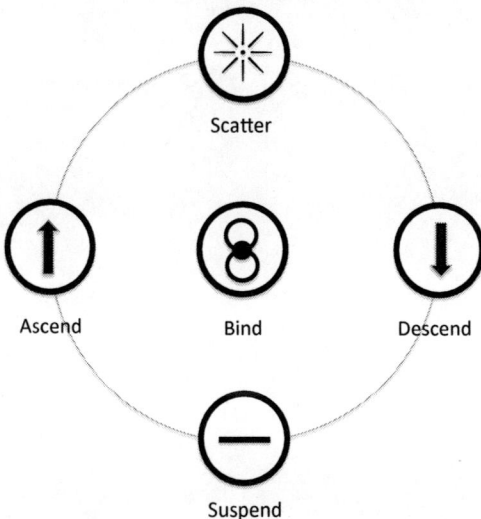

Scatter

Ascend   Bind   Descend

Suspend

Together these five movements represent aspects of our consciousness and form a kind of "mind map" that clinicians can use in approaching emotional disorders. Below is a brief summary of the five movements and purposes of qi as reflected in sensory perceptions and emotional expressions. I have found this to be an invaluable tool to help gain deeper understanding of what a child's emotional symptoms are trying to accomplish. From this we can develop holistic strategies to empower each child express his or her Big Heartedness.

The Five Phases of Emotions Chart

Ⓘ Ascending	✳ Scattering	Ⓑ Binding	Ⓓ Descending	⊖ Suspending
Wood	**Fire**	**Earth**	**Metal**	**Water**
Spring	Summer	Harvest	Autumn	Winter
Liver	Heart	Spleen	Lung	Kidney
Locomotion	Circulation	Digestion	Respiration	Restoration
Purpose:	Purpose:	Purpose:	Purpose:	Purpose:
When too still	When too much	When too	When too	When too
or too low-	thrust-	expanded-	bound-	distinct-
To rise up	To lighten up	To contain	To refine	To stop
To move	To expand	To collect	To define	To settle
forward	To illuminate	To recollect	To untangle	To still
To free up	To excite	To connect	To cut down	To deepen
To see ahead	To awaken	To combine	To sort	To reflect
Big Hearted Ascending:	Big Hearted Scattering:	Big Hearted Binding:	Big Hearted Descending:	Big Hearted Suspending:
Heroic	Joy	Thoughtfulness	Ethical	Wisdom
Perseverance	Delight	Kindness	Judgment	Curiosity
Dignity	Compassion	Humanity	Aesthetic	Reflection
Determination	Humor	Contextual	precision	Creativity
Courage	Spectacle	understanding	Justice	Imagination
Encouragement	Transcendence	Loyalty	Temperance	
Insecure Ascending:	Insecure Scattering:	Insecure Binding:	Insecure Descending:	Insecure Suspending
Hyperactivity	Impulsivity	Obsessive	Disappointed	Apathetic
Aggression	Panic attacks	worry	Depressed	Negativistic
Low frustration	Distracted	No boundaries	Compulsive	Fatalistic
Conduct	Dramatic mood	Indecisive	Ritualistic	Immobilized by
disorder	shifts	"Knotted"	Loss of	fear
Defiant	Hysteria	Needy	spontaneity	Oppositional
Somatic:	Somatic:	Somatic:	Somatic:	Somatic:
Tension	Palpitations	Stomachaches	Constipation	Low back pain
headache	Reflux	Indigestion	Asthma	Adrenal fatigue
Muscle twitch	Explosive	Leaky gut	Eczema	Arthritis
hypertension	diarrhea	Easy bruising	Tics	

©cowan 2012

There are intimate relationships between these five movements and directions that proceed like the cycle of seasons. Each serves the heart in manifesting one's destiny by promoting growth and development and providing counterbalance to other motions and emotions (see five phase diagram below). Just as one season is not necessarily better than the others, there is no hierarchy within these movements, one may simply be more effective in certain conditions. It is only when these movements manifest in excessive or insufficient ways that balance to the whole is thrown off.

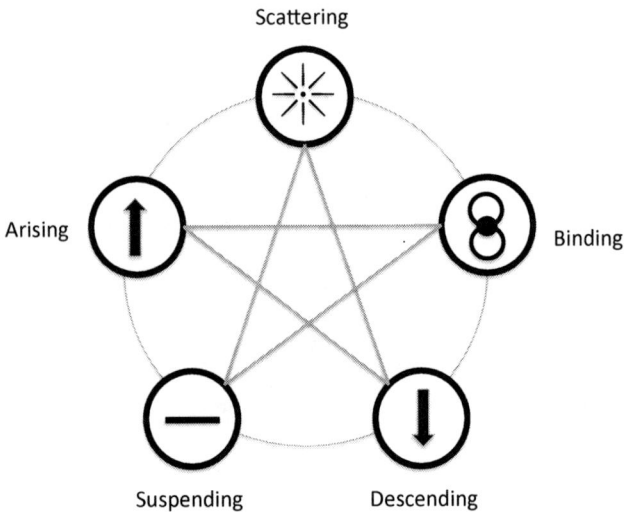

Each child has something to offer the world. A child has a specific style of resonating that corresponds to what attracts or distract her. These driving forces are linked to her destiny and what she is here to teach us. This is invaluable information for practitioners who are interested in creating individualized treatment strategies. Our goal is to help each child become a virtuoso of her emotions in the world. It is important when working with emotions in children to pay close attention to the quality and direction of these emotions and ask yourself what the movement is trying to accomplish.

For example, David is a child who is prone to easy frustration and intense anger outbursts, lashing out at the smallest provocation. This represents the ascending movement of qi. Ascending qi corresponds to the movement of spring, the force of the stem pushing through the ground and the Wood phase. Emerging from the suspended animation of winter, there is a natural power to rise up and confront boundaries, to find freedom from constraints, to move forward towards the promise of something better. It reflects a specific movement in response to feelings of inferiority or oppression. Rising qi allows one to feel superior. Its virtue lies in being able to rise up in dignity, to see the path ahead and get the job done. When driven by Big Heartedness, this particular adaptive style is reflected in qualities like heroic perseverance, decision-making and noble leadership. But when this tendency to ascend comes from an insecure base, it can result in excessive psychological disturbances such as hostility, aggression, hyperactivity, paranoia and conduct disorders. Because the mind and body are aspects of one organism, such exaggerated movements of qi may also manifest somatically as tension headaches, stiff neck and hypertension.

Working with a child like David begins by first identifying the feelings behind these emotions and helping the child embrace the secret Wood powers hidden within these feeling. As David learned to identify with his primary secret powers, we began training in recovering his true strengths of character. For a Wood child, for example, this requires creating settings that offer brief opportunities to experience calm (represented by Water-Suspend). In Five Phase dynamics, Water nourishes Wood (just as winter become spring). When a Wood child practices experiencing calm moments, he can begin to suspend his actions and simply reflect on the feelings without judgment before and after they become emotions and behaviors. This is how David began to notice what recovery actually feels like. By offering a structured environment where David could practice exercises like breathing and begin labeling feeling (Metal-Descend), he was able to gain more confidence in defining what he perceived with greater accuracy and without being threatened. This creates some space between the intensity of feeling and emoting-behaving for him to explore the subtler shades of emotions. Eventually he could say "I'm just a little angry." This is a hallmark of recovery. It is important to explain to parents that this process takes time. Working with parents to recognize their own natural propensities to react is critically important in developing a wholehearted family approach. Offering activities that encourage the Wood Child to be a role model allowed David to extend his secret powers for the good of others (Fire-Scatter). In David's case, becoming a performer had a powerful effect on his ability to regulate his emotions more effectively. Eventually, he was able to identify his own feelings with those of others and rather than simply pushing his agenda, become a true hero to his peers through the power of empathy and kindness (Earth-Binding). Through this process, David's parents discovered creative ways to empower him to maintain connection to the clarity of his Big Heart and truly manifest his destiny.

Nature Favors Diversity

Each child resonates within a specific set of adaptive styles. They are gifts to our world. The key to our creativity and survival as a species rests in our natural diversity of talents and expressions. Expecting all children to respond in exactly the same way to circumstances is, to say the least, unnatural and dangerous. When we deny our diversity, we are forced to constrain our expressions and suppress our emotions. This leads to a vicious cycle of chronic pathology.

In teaching children and their parents to become more aware of the direction of their feelings, they learn how to shape their natural predispositions into more effective contributions to the world. Chinese Medicine has developed a powerful method of understanding how each of the five adaptive styles: *wood*, *fire*, *earth*, *metal* and *water* influence each other. This system of spiritual ecology generates practical ways to enhance each child's emotional resilience and wellbeing. Emotions are contagious. When we as caregivers feel our children's emotions as cries for help rather than something broken, we develop our own big hearts. These become the healing emotions that with imagination and compassion empower our children to resonate in wholehearted ways with the natural processes of life, and in doing so we are actively participating in shaping the future health of our world.

(Endnotes)

1 Hinshaw S. 2005 The stigmatization of mental illness in children and parents: developmental issues, family concerns and research needs. Journal of child psychol. 46:7 pp 714-734

2 The Harvard Medical Letter 2007 May Bipolar disorder in children

3 Greenberg, M. Promoting resilience in Children and youth: preventive interventions and their interface with neuroscience 2006

4 Szyf, M. The epigenetic impact of early life adversity 2009

5 Ainsworth M. et al 1978. Patterns of Attachment. Hillsdale, NJ: Erlbaum.

6 Dimassio, A. 1999 The feeling of what happens: body, emotion and the making of consciousness.

7 Moffitt, TE et al. 2011 A gradient of childhood self-control predicts health, ealth and public safety. PNAS 108 (7): 2693-2698

8 Cowan, S. 2012, Fire Child Water Child, how understanding the five types of ADHD can help you improve your child's self-esteem and attention.

Appendix B

All Disease Comes From the Heart: The Pivotal Role of the Emotions in Classical Chinese Medicine

by Heiner Fruehauf, PhD. L.Ac.

Most modern clinicians find that a majority of their patients suffer from the symptom complex generally referred to as "stress". Emotional stress, however, is usually regarded as a confounding rather than a causative factor in pathophysiology. This assessment is contrary to the tenets of classical Chinese medicine, which originally regarded emotional imbalance as a spiritual affliction of primary significance. While ancient Chinese philosophy considered emotional sensibility as our greatest asset in the process of fulfilling human destiny, it also regarded human temperaments as our greatest liability due to vast pathogenetic potential.

While Western medicine has encountered psychosomatic theory in the 20th century, the subtle and non-quantifiable nature of the emotions continues to be viewed as a nebulous factor by the purveyors of materialist science. The result is that modern physicians generally ignore or medicate symptoms of stress, depression or anxiety. This bias has affected how institutionalized -Chinese medicine views the topic of the emotions today. While the contemporary brand of Chinese medicine, exported by the People's Republic of China under the trade name "TCM", acknowledges that the treatment of non-local and non-structural symptoms belongs to its therapeutic domain, textbook TCM theory lacks both a cohesive and in-depth approach to the nature and dynamics of human feelings.

Through a review of relevant ancient sources, this essay intends to heighten awareness about the original complexity and significance that classical Chinese medicine bestowed on the subject of the emotions. Written more than 2,000 years ago, many of the texts cited below remind us that most diseases in urban human beings are caused by emotional stress. This is pertinent clinical advice that more than ever applies to the realities of contemporary Chinese medicine practice.

The Relationship of Body and Spirit

"I believe that there are two different human methodologies of knowing: one is time oriented, and the other is space oriented." (1) Thus begins an analysis of the differences between Chinese medicine and modern science by the contemporary philosopher Liu Changlin. He goes on to describe how Chinese medicine is time therapy, based in the ancient science of energy dynamics, while Western medicine is space therapy, rooted in the modern science of matter analysis. Indeed, the major distinction between modern and ancient physicians is how they viewed the nature and relationship of matter, energy, and consciousness. What came first, the chicken or the egg? All medicines rooted in scientific materialism as well as Marxist materialism answer resoundingly in favor of matter. It is no accident that the modern Chinese term for psycho-somatic is *xing-shen bingxue*, literally the science of how (primary) physical form and (secondary) spirit relate in the disease forming process. A 1991 TCM primer on body-mind connections elaborates: "In the relationship of matter (*xing)* and spirit *(shen)*, matter takes the leading role, while the phenomena of the mind and the emotions are secondary to it; first there is matter, then there is consciousness; consciousness is born of matter." (2) Within this paradigm, the philosopher Xunzi is generally regarded as a pioneer of "progressive materialist thinking", while most Buddhist and Taoist texts on the subject matter are identified as "idealist musings, spawned by the backward conditions of China's feudal past." (3)

In contrast to this position, the defining classics of Chinese medicine establish that it is the invisible forces of *shen* (spirit) and *qi* (functional force) that rule matter. "Heaven comes first", asserts the *Lingshu*, "earth is second". (4) Or in the more elaborate words of Liu Zhou, a 6th century philosopher: "If the spirit is at peace, the heart is in harmony; when the heart is in harmony, the body is whole; if the spirit becomes aggravated the heart wavers, and when the heart wavers the spirit becomes injured; if one seeks to heal the physical body, therefore, one needs to regulate the spirit first." (5) Following the premise of one of Chinese medicine's most fundamental tenets, *jing-qi-shen* theory (the Chinese forerunner of body-mind-spirit theory), Chinese medical diagnosis aims primarily at determining the condition of *qi* and *shen*, while Chinese medical therapy endeavors to treat *qi* and *shen*. This includes situations where the primary goal is to affect changes in the physical body. The central Chinese medicine concept of *shen* appearing in early Chinese texts could conceivably be summarized as "that which is subtle and invisible, yet commands everything."

One of the topics woven through all of the major medical classics- the *Yellow Emperor's Classic of Medicine* (Neijing), the *Classic of Difficulties* (Nanjing), and the *Treatise on Disorders Caused by Cold and Miscellaneous Syndromes* (Shanghan zabing lun)-- is the concept of the superior physician (*shanggong*). According to all of these sources, it is the defining characteristic of a preeminent healer to be able to diagnose and treat diseases on the *shen* level. The *Neijing* states in an exemplary line: "The superior physician makes it his prerogative to treat disease when it has not yet structurally manifested, and prevents being in the position of having to treat disorders that have already progressed to the realm of the physical." (6) In contrast, "the low level physician finds himself salvaging what has already manifested in physical form, and treating what is already ruined." (7) The top-level physician thus perceives what the average practitioner cannot see:

The physical body- yes, you need to work with it when your eyes cannot perceive, by asking where the discomfort is and by palpating the channels... *Shen*, on the other hand, yes *shen*-in order to diagnose on this level you need not be focused on what the patient tells you. Your eyes see the invisible, your heart is open, and your intuitive sensing is front and center. All of a sudden, then, the subtle truth will reveal itself to you, without being able to put your experience into words, seeing while everybody else does not; as if the night turns bright for you alone while everybody else remains in the dark, like the invisible hand of the wind moving the clouds. That is why it is called *shen*, mysterious. (8)

An exemplary doctor, therefore, follows the tenets of ancient times, experiences their magic in the present, keeps the inner eye on the subtle and mysterious, and stays connected to the realm of the unlimited- what the pack does not see is what the excellent physician values;... that is why the superior physician works with the invisible sprouts when grasping *qi*, while the inferior physician is mired in the realm of what has already become manifest, thereby contributing to the decline of the body." (9) The priorities of a classical Chinese medicine practitioner are thus summarized as follows: "One, treat the spirit; two, know how to nourish the physical body; three, know the true transmission of herbal medicine; four, work with the large and small types of needles; and five, know how to diagnose the state of *qi* and blood in the *fu* and *zang* organs." (10)

Between Heaven and Earth: Human Destiny and the Heart

In 1174, the Song dynasty scholar-physician Chen Yan re-capped three general causes for disease *(sanyin)* that still serve as a model for Chinese medical pathogenesis:

> The first category is called internal causes, refer-ring to the seven emotions *(qiqing)* that emerge from the organ systems inside and then reflect as structural pathology in the body's outer regions; the next is called external causes, referring to the six excessive weather influences *(liuyin)* that invade the channels and collaterals from the outside and in due course end up lodging in the organ systems; the last is called not internal not external causes, referring to injuries to the vital force from eating too little or too much food, or by bites from tigers, wolves, and poisonous insects, as well as accidents involving weapons, drowning and the like. (11)

While Chen's work generally gets credited with the in-troduction of "the theory of the three causes", the charac-terization of emotional versus non-emotional pathology is as old as the Chinese notion of disease itself. Beginning with the earliest medical texts, two Chinese characters are generally used to describe the concept of disease, namely *ji* and *bing*. An early dictionary defines *ji* as "an acute disease that arises when alien *qi* strikes a person from the outside." (12) In contrast, the more common term *bing* is described as "a more severe and complex disease" (13) that "is attached to a person's righteous *qi* inside the body". (14) On the most literal level, *bing* means "affliction of the heart". It consists of a combination of the disease radical (originally a pictogram of a bedridden person) and the heavenly stem *bing*, which is associated with the phase element fire and the heart organ. Together, the complete character signifies a situation where somebody has become physically ill due to mental, emotional, or spiritual causes. (15)

Despite this unequivocal portrayal of the leading role of *shen* and its pivotal part in the disease forming process, contemporary TCM has banished the role of the emotions to the historical archives of Chinese medicine, along with many other aspects of classical Chinese medicine that do not mesh with the ideology of Marxist materialist science. Consequently, many modern Chinese medical practitioners tend to pay more attention to viruses and bacteria than to emotional stress as causative factors of disease.

In contrast to this recent development, all eminent physicians of the past agreed that only animals and enlightened sages are capable of escaping the influence of the emotions, while the average human being is susceptible to their pathogenetic potential. The 18th century physician Xu Dachun once remarked, "The treatment of humans should differ from that of animals, because animal diseases are rarely caused by emotional factors, but by wind, cold, and food related problems." (16) As if augmenting this statement, Miu Xiyong pointed out in 1625: "In very ancient antiquity, human illness was primarily caused by the six excessive weather patterns rather than the seven emotions. Today, the situation is quite different- the seven emotional influences are severe and the five desires run deep." (17)

Feelings and emotions, therefore, are at the core of the human condition- defined by ancient Chinese sources as the plight of having been given a heart, a heart that keeps the human being suspended in the dynamic struggle between the earthy demons of the animal body and the virtuous spirits of his/her heavenly nature. The *Shuowen jiezi*, China's earliest dictionary, defines the heart as "the human heart; it is the earth organ". (18) In addition to distinguishing the complexities of the human spirit from other living things, this remarkable 2nd century statement makes reference to a little known fact: in the early stages of Chinese medicine the heart was alternately classified as the earth organ, not the fire organ that it is exclusively described as today. From the perspective of Chinese cosmology, it seems only appropriate that the heart- the 'empty vessel' and container of *shen*- was first described as an earthen receptacle. Similar to the story of creation that appears in the Old Testament as well as other ancient traditions, Chinese mythology conveys that humans were first made from clay: People say that when Heaven and earth opened and unfolded, humankind did not yet exist. Nu Gua (the creatrix) kneaded yellow earth and fashioned human beings." (19) The human condition, therefore, is metaphorically described as the state of having an earthen heart, which in its healthy state is capable of containing the fire of spirit, including the emotions and their potentially troublesome ramifications.

Another common denominator that relates the heart to the phase element earth and the evolving fate of humanity is the number five. Multiple ancient texts, including the *Neijing*, relate or make reference to the theory that all life forms are divided into five categories: the scaly creatures, signified by the water element and the number 1 (representative: dragon), the winged creatures, signified by the fire element and the number 2 (representative: phoenix); the furry creatures, signified by the wood element and the number three (representative: unicorn); the armored creatures, signified by the metal element and the number 4 (representative: turtle); the naked creatures, signified by the earth element and the number 5 (representative: human being or, in some sources, the sage). (20)

From an ancient Chinese perspective, humans quite literally tick to the rhythm of five. The *Guanzi*, a text attributed to the philopher Guan Zhong who lived during the 7th century B.C.E., observes that "the human being completes physical form after five lunar months and is born after ten." (21) Five represents the union of the first yang number 3 and the first yin number 2, and is described by many ancient traditions as the number of the ultimate sentiment- love. Five, as yang joining and moving within yin, is thus the numerical rendition of earth containing fire, or spirit moving within the body. This is perhaps the main reason why Chinese medical theory features the five phase element system as the primary means to diagnose the human being. It is the most suitable system to assess the flow of "humanity": the flow of divine spirit within the matter of the animal body.

The number five is inextricably associated with the five phases and thus with movement itself, harmonizing the upward momentum of earth with the downward momentum of heaven. The human heart, appropriately associated with the 5th month of the lunar cycle, is primarily earth and secondarily fire. A major part of being human means to come to terms with the nature of this clay: a dense clod with beastly memories, yet with a heaven-bound mission that is paralleled by the evolution of human posture. While most animals walk on four legs manifesting their earthly destiny, humans walk upright with their head pointed skyward, fulfilling a destiny that includes the discovery of heaven within earth. Five, therefore, is both the number of humanity and evolution. To the creators of Chinese medicine, being human meant to be endowed with a heart and the resultant potential to sense, connect to, and ritually celebrate the higher dimensions regarded as the source of all life. The ever moving and reactive nature of the human heart, however, requires that in this process the fickleness of fire is contained by the stability of earth. Otherwise, the spirit becomes ungrounded, opening the door for the seven emotions to unfold their consumptive effects.

****

The Power of Ritual and the Emotional Therapy

System of the Confucian Educator Wang Fengyi (1864-1937)

"The difference of being in command and losing command over the emotions is the root of life and death, and the starting point of living and dying." (22) Thus the *Annals of Master Lu* sums up conventional Chinese wisdom regarding the quandary of human feelings, stressing that mastery of one's emotions is a requirement for maintaining health and longevity. The same source also reveals the now well-known medical fact that emotional imbalance initiates energetic stagnation, a potential cause for phlegm, blood stasis, and other harbingers of structural pathology. To resolve the acute discomfort brought on by emotional stress and depression, modern Chinese medicine practitioners commonly prescribe herbal remedies such as Xiaoyao San, the famous 11th century "powder for dispersing stuck emotions and restoring leisure and ease." However, many physicians of the past believed that the deeper strata of emotional injury cannot be treated with herbs, but need to be addressed by affecting the spirit directly. Xu Dachun, for instance, describes how to employ the controlling cycle of the phase elements to treat disease originating from excess emotional indulgence:

> If the five sentiments have been strongly injured, this condition cannot be treated with herbs, but should be addressed via the controlling relationship cycle. Grief controls anger, use it to touch an angry

person with tales of misery and dejection; excitement controls grief, use it to thrill a sad person by inundating him with waves of sarcasm and degrading language; fear can control excitement, use it to intimidate a maniacal person with threats of death and imminent disaster; anger can control worry, use it to trigger a depressed person with foul and shameful language; worry can control fear, use it to approach a panicky person with depressing news of potential loss. (23)

While this approach of "treating fire with fire" has also been reported in the clinical case histories of other physicians, it represents by no means a widely accepted cure for imbalanced emotions. More typically, some of the religious sources call for an outright "elimination" and "rejection" of the emotions, while most texts prescribe a more moderate approach, advocating the balancing of strong feelings by channeling them in appropriate ways. The key word used in this context is *jie* (to harmonize, to moderate, to create rhythm). Many of the relevant texts define moderation as a distinct quality of the sages, who alone are said to be capable of using emotions appropriately, to achieve deep connection without being led astray and eventually succumbing to illness. For the average person, the best way to moderate the agitated spirit is the institution of rituals, as the famous 1st century historian Ban Gu explains in the following passage:

The human being contains both the yin and the yang influences of Heaven and earth, and consequently manifests the emotions of partiality, hate, excitement, anger, sorrow, and pleasure; hence, the divisive nature of humanity which is so hard to moderate. The sages alone are capable of moderating this aspect of the human condition, and thus created ritual and music guided by the example of Heaven and earth, using them to stay connected to the all-governing light of spirit, establishing the laws of human behavior, straightening out the relationship between human nature and the emotions, and thus achieving moderation in the myriad affairs of life. For the feelings between a man and a woman and the sensation of jealousy, they created the ritual of marriage; for the social interactions between elders and younger members of the community, they created the ritual of celebratory banquets; for the feelings of grieving the dead and missing loved ones, they created the ritual of sacrificial mourning; for the desire to venerate one's leaders, they created the ritual of audience. A mourning ritual features ritual wailing and stomping, while music has a set format for dances and songs- sufficient to warm the sentiments of the straight, and to prevent missteps by those who are crooked. If the ritual of marriage gets abandoned, then the Tao of husband and wife will become lacking, and consequently the sins of sexual decadence and abstinence will increase; if the ritual of celebratory banquets gets abandoned, then the proper order between the older and younger generations will be lost, and the crimes of quarreling and flattery will blossom; if the ritual of mourning and burial gets abandoned, then the gratitude we owe our own flesh and blood becomes weak, and many of the dead will forget about the living; if the ritual of audience gets abandoned, the the proper position of ruler and servant becomes confused, and war and turmoil will generally arise. (24)

According to the system of the five natures/virtues introduced in an earlier section of this article, *li* (propriety, sacred connection, ritual) is the function most directly associated with the heart. As a scholar of Chinese medicine, it was most interesting for me to uncover this explicit connection between emotional healing and ancient Chinese ritual, a topic usually thought of as the musty turf of anthropologists and religious historians. It further strengthened the conviction first imparted to me by most of my older Chinese mentors that meaningful resesarch on the foundational concepts of Oriental medicine requires an immersion in the textual environment of *Neijing* and pre-*Neijing* times.

From a clinical perspective, the concept of propriety, ritual, and moderated emotions is admittedly as popular today as wearing great-aunt Bertha's dress on a Saturday night out in town. It was thus an illuminating experience for me to encounter a group of Northern Chinese therapists who still use the Confucian teachings of virtue, ritual, and social relationship as their primary treatment tool. Their approach to healing is radical, especially when considering the fact that they are practicing in the territory of the People's Republic of China- their work is ostensibly devoid of pharmaceuticals, herbs or needles, but exclusively uses the non-material methods of storytelling and ritual affirmation. Echoing some of the ancient sources introduced earlier, these practitioners believe that most diseases originate from a darkening of the bright aspects of human nature by the veil of inappropriate emotions.

The origins of this healing modality- still practiced widely in the Northern provinces of Liaoning, Jilin, and Heilongjiang- are rooted in the teachings of Wang Fengyi, a Confucian educator and charismatic emotional healer who was extremely influential in this part of China during the early part of the 20th century. Wang's biography relates that he grew up as a poor and illiterate peasant, and became enlightened to the nature of human emotions and their disease-causing consequences while observing the traditional three-year watch over his father's grave. (25) He observed that all emotions arise from social interactions, especially within the nucleus of community relationship, one's immediate family. Driven by an urgent sense of mission to help save his community from the curse of disease amidst the misery of poverty and civil war, he began traveling from village to village, spreading a neo-Confucian version of everyday-life spirituality focusing on proper family relationships. His oral presentations, some of them preserved in the form of reprinted lecture excerpts, were legendary at the time, drawing largely from rural audiences. Many participants were reported to be crying, fainting, or vomiting when triggered into a state of recognition and ruefulness by the transmission of the master.

In addition, Wang Fengyi greatly contributed to the revolutionary movement of bringing education to Chinese women. He was instrumental in establishing and maintaining seven hundred schools for girls, since he considered it to be a shortcoming of traditional Confucian doctrine that women were not entitled to an education. Wang's philosophy of self-responsibility viewed the roles of women (mothers, wives, daughters-in-law) as the central element for the health of every family member as well as the country at large. He felt, moreover, that women were best able to exemplify the core essence of his social philosophy, namely the virtue of giving compassion to others while reserving severity for oneself. In this sense, Wang looms large as a modern transmitter of the teachings of Confucius, Dong Zhongshu, and Zhu Xi. Many of Wang's teachings, as well as those of his students, sound remarkably like the following passage written by Dong Zhongshu in the 2nd century BCE:

> What the *Annals* are teaching us to regulate is how to deal with others. How to deal with the self and how to deal with others is exemplified by the virtues of compassion and selflessness. With compassion, we make others feel good, while with selflessness, we set the self straight; that is why compassion

is associated with others, and selflessness with self...
Compassion is manifested by loving others, not by
loving self; selflessness is manifested by straightening out the self, not by straightening out others.
(26)

From the perspective of Chinese medicine, it is the elaborate system of five element associations that is the most
significant part of Wang's legacy. This system contains the
familiar relations of the five phase elements with the five
organs, the five colors, the five smells, etc., but synthesizes
them with the ancient teachings on human virtue as well
as Wang's own remarkable insights and experiences as a
therapist. Now as then, patients are generally asked to relate
their stories and then are diagnosed with a specific breach
of virtue caused by one of the five emotional poisons,
specifically anger (wood), hate (fire), blame (earth), judgment (metal), or disdain (water). While Wang himself was
known to be an exceptionally clairvoyant healer and some
of his students maintain this gift, for the denser minded he
has left behind detailed descriptions of how affliction in
different body parts may be related to specific emotions and
specific family members.

The curative process of Wang's system involves the therapist's weaving a narrative, ranging from very few words to
night-long marathons of storytelling that are able to "turn
the heart of the patient". The material for stories is often
taken from the treasure trove of Chinese moral history, but
most typically involve the daily environment of the patient:

stories of Master Wang curing someone just like them, or vivid tales of the cure or demise of someone in the next village, or ideally, someone present in the room or the village square who offers heart-wrenching and tearful testimony of their own healing process. This method is referred to as *xingli jiangbing*, literally "talking the disease away by appealing to one's higher nature". The curative effect is considered to begin when the patient is moved to acknowledge his own emotional involvement in the disease forming process, and commits to transform his/her blame toward others into a thorough reformation of self. At this point, which skillful storytellers are sometimes able to trigger in minutes while others may need days or even weeks, the patient typically begins to vomit into ready-made buckets, or exhibits other signs of physical cleansing such as crying, sweating, or diarrhea. One of the healers I visited remarked matter-of-factly that "liver cirrhosis can be disgorged in one week, while with some cancers it takes three weeks or longer until no more tar-like materials are being brought up".

Transcripts of these healing sessions may often read flat, especially to someone who originates from a different cultural background, but both healers and patients insist that it is the transmission from the storyteller herself- achieved by a non-compromised lifestyle of virtuous conduct- that is needed to trigger a powerful response. Through modern eyes, the nature of these healing sessions may look similar to the phenomenon of the *qigong baogao* (Qigong transmission lecture) which were so common in China before the official crackdown on Falun Gong practitioners. By virtue of their humble demeanor and their radically selfless conduct, however, the talk-practitioners of the Manchurian plains tend to cut a different figure than the entrepreneurial Qigong masters of the 1990's. In the particularly moving example of the peasant healer I saw in a village near the Russian border, his simple house had been converted into a make-shift hospice where deathly ill patients traveled to from far away and stayed for free, were fed for free, and received treatment for free- day afer day for the last twenty-five years, sometimes adding up to 20-40 people per day. Prior to receiving permission from his mentor to start the practice of therapeutic storytelling, moreover, he had to spend twenty years preparing for this work by first clearing his own emotional issues.

Last summer, I had the privilege of spending one week with healers of Wang Fengyi's lineage, and was able to directly witness the intense process of storytelling and ensuing physical cleansing. While this was far too little time to verify many of the miraculous outcomes that this method of treatment is said to have achieved during the last century, including the complete cure of diabetes, aplastic anemia, congenital heart disease, and many types of cancer, it is my distinct impression as a medical professional that I witnessed something very profound, existing in the present moment and on a relatively large scale. As a scholar of the foundational theory of classical Chinese medicine, moreover, I marvel at how completely the ancient system of emotional pathology and therapy has survived in this lineage, and how relevant it is still today.

In conclusion, I feel that the ancient Chinese theory on the emotions offers another example of the profundity of ancient medical theories. Confucius himself once emphasized, "He who by reanimating the Old can gain knowledge of the New is fit to be a teacher". (27) Wang Fengyi and his students have demonstrated that no matter how antiquated or out-dated an ancient concept may look, truly classical knowledge is timeless and has the capacity of being fiercely relevant for the present. I hope that this essay can serve as a beginning step in clarifying some of the confusion surrounding the theory of the emotions in Chinese medicine, as well as inspire some relevant clinical insights.

Endnotes

1) See Liu Changlin, "Fazhan zhongyixue de guanjian" (How to Develop the Core Essence of Chinese Medicine), in Zheyan kan zhongyi (Chinese Medicine Seen through Philosopher's Eyes) (Beijing: Beijing Kexue Jishu Chubanshe, 2005), pp. 28-34; English translation by Heiner Fruehauf viewable at www.classicalchinesemedicine.org

2) See Dong Lianrong et.al., ed., Zhongyi xingshen bing xue (Body-Mind Relationships in Chinese Medicine) (Beijing: Guangming Ribao Chubanshe, 1991), p. 3

3) Ibid., p. 1

4) See chapter 78 of the Lingshu, in guo Xiechun,

ed., Huangdi neijing lingshu (The Yellow Emperor's Classic of Medicine: The Spiritual Pivot) (Tianjin: Tianjin Kexue Jishu Chubanshe) p. 514

5)   See chapter 1 on the Liuzi (Master Liu), in Raizi quanshu (A Complete Collection of Works by the One Hundred Masters) 8 vols. (Shanghai Zhejiang Renmin Chubanshe, 1991), vol. 6, p. 1

6)   See chapter 2 of the Suwen, in Nanjing Zhongyi Xueyuan, ed., Huangdi neijing suwen yishi (An Annotated Text With Translation of the Yellow Emperor's Classic of Medicine: Plain Questions) (Shanghai: Shanghai Kexue Jishu Chubanshe, 1991), p. 16; see a similar version of this quote in chapter 55 of the Lingshu, in Huangdi neijing lingshu, p. 379

7)   See chapter 26 of the Suwen, in Huangdi neijing suwen yishi, p. 204

8)   Ibid., p. 206

9)   See chapter 73 of the Lingshu, in Huangdi neijing lingshu, p. 473

10) See chapter 25 of the Suwen, in Huangdi neijing suwen yishi, p. 198

11) See the Siku quanshu introduction to Chen Yan, Sanyin jiyi bingzheng fanglun (Analysis and Formulas for Same Diseases Generated by the Three Causes); in Yan Shiyun, ed., Zhongguo yiji tongkao (A Comprehensive Analysis of Chinese Medical Books), 4 vols. (Shanghai: Shanghai Zhongyi Xueyuan Chubanshe, 1992), vol. 2, p. 2239

12) See Shiming (An Explication of Terms), quoted on Zhang Liwei et al, ed., Kangxi zidian tongjie (A Comprehensive Explanation of the Kangxi Dictionary), 3 vols. (Changchun: Shida Wenyi Chubanshe, 1997), vol. 2, p. 1392

13) See Xu Shen, and Tang Kejing, annotator, Shuowen jiezi jinshi (A Modern Annotated Version of Elucidating Lines and Explaining Complex Characters), 2 vols. (Changsha: Qiuli Shushe, 2002), vol. 1, p. 1016

14) She Shiming, quoted in Kangxi zidian tongjie, vol 2, p. 1393

15) See also Liu Lihong's interpretation of the character bing, in Liu Lihong, Kikao zhongyi (Contemplating Chinese Medicine) (Guilin: Guangxi Shifan Daxue Chubanshe, 2003), pp. 151-53

16) See Xu Dachun, "Shouyi lun" (A Discussion of Veterinary Medicine) in his Yixue yuanliu lun (A Treatise on the Source Traditions of Medicine), in vol. 2 of the Siku quanshu edition, no page numbers

17) See Miu Xiyong, "Yaoxing zhuzhi canhu zhigui" (A Reference Guide to the Nature and Therapeutic Effect of Herbs), in his Shen Nong bencao jing shu (An Annotated Version of Shen Nong's Materia Medica), in vol 1 of the Siku quanshu edition, no page numbers

18) See Shuowen jiezi jinshi, vol. 2, p. 1438

19) See the Han dynasty text Fengsu tongyi (Explanations of Social Customs), translated in Anne

Birrell, Chinese Mythology: An Introduction (Baltimore: Johns Hopkins University Press, 1993) p. 35

20) See, for instance, the Da Dai liji (the Elder Dai's Record of Ritual); in the Neijing suwen, this concept is referred to in chapters 67 and 70.

21) See chapter 39 of the Guanzi (Master Guan), in Baizi quanshu, vol. 3, no page numbers (for third section of article and footnotes, go to www.classicalchinesemedicine.org)

22) See chapter 2 of Lushi chumqiui, in Baizi Quanshu, vol.4, no page numbers

23) See Xu Dachun, "Wai nei jun xiang pian," in Chishui xuanzhu in vo. 1 of the Siku quanshu edition, no page numbers

24) See Hanshu (history of the Former Han, quoted in Xun Rui, Qian Han Ji (A Record of the Former Han) vol. 5 of the Siku quanshu edition, no page numbers

25) See Wang Fengyi nianpu yu yulu (A Biographic Table of Events in Wang Fengyi's life and Record of his Oral Teachings) (no publisher, 2000) Note that most of the numerous publications on Wang Fengyi's teachings are reproduced and circulated by tight knit Buddhist or Confucian circles and are generally not for sale to the public.

26) See chapter 8 of the Chunqiu fanlu, Siku quanshu edition, no page numbers

27) See Aruthur Waley, tr., Confucius: The Ana-

lects (London: Everyman's Library, 2000), p. 82

Virtues

by Thea Elijah, LAc

The Five Element perspective is not very focused on illness. If you ask a 5 E practitioner where the person got that headache or to do an analysis of a particular symptom, we're pretty feeble with coming up with an analysis of illness. If you ask us to describe what is this client's health, what is their potential, what are they actually going for, what would they look like when they're well, we're much more likely to have something powerful to say because what we're working with is understanding how natural energies move through different kinds of people, and what that looks like when it is flourishing.

JR Worseley always talked about how, in order to treat someone, you have to be able to see who they would be if they were well. Not necessarily in detail, but a general feeling. The 5 Elements perspective is designed to help us with exactly this. We can tell what the 'true' note would be by what the 'off' note sounds like. In other words, if the client is manifesting all sorts of pathologies of the Wood element, then we know their health is going to be a healthy Wood element. We have a sense of what Springtime and vigorously growing plants are like. The quality of the illness implies the nature of the health, like the flip side of a coin. An ill tomato plant implies the flourishing tomato plant. An ill palm tree implies the flourishing palm tree. We're looking at using the patterns of nature, as seen in the ill person, to be able to resonate with and draw forth a person's journey to wholeness and beyond.

As an organic vegetable farmer, it's very clear to me, you can spend all your time trying to get rid of the bugs. Or, you can nourish the plants, give them what they need for their flourishing, and you know what? The bugs are gone. You don't have to think about the bugs so much if you're giving this plant what it needs. But, what does *this* plant need versus what *that* plant needs? What are the needs for thriving of different beings? That's the central question from a 5 E perspective, what are the needs for thriving of this part of nature, this creature, this organism in front of me. This is what the 5E diagnostic system is to determine.

What will it take for this being to thrive? It will be a different recipe for different kinds of people; not everyone's health is the same! Metal people need order and rhythm. Fire people need more spontaneity. Wood people need to know what the Road Map is. 'Where are we headed?'

There are many different ways of thriving. This is described by the 5E Transformations of virtue, which are the ways of taking our wobbles as entry point to thriving.

What's the difference between the infant and the sage, both of which are perfect embodiments of *de (*virtue)? The sage is an infant who grew up and got completely messed up just like the rest of us, and then found her way back home again- and, in the process, gained self-aware consciousness. Both the infant and the sage have this virtue of authentic spontaneous self becoming, but the infant has no awareness. The sage does, and yet is able to remain just as authentic and spontaneous as the infant. The journey from infant to sage is something like this: we're with the Tao, we fall from the Tao, and we make our way back again. Which way we fell (or have an ongoing tendency to fall, which is what generates illness) has something to do with which way we're going to come back.

For the most part, my interest in working diagnostically with the 5E and with the Virtues is to work with them nonverbally, because I know more from my body and from the client's response in their body whether or not I'm on track. My primary influences in really good psycho-spiritual work are 5 Element veterinarians. 5 Element veterinarians never get caught up in the client's story. When a veterinarian establishes rapport, it's not by talking to them about what their mother did or didn't do. It's all body language. It's all tone of voice. Both from the practitioner and from the animal. It's easy to get caught up in projecting psychological ideas onto our clients. Physical expressions of distress or ease are more reliable.

A tremendous amount of communication is nonverbal. How can we be in our bodies in ways that resonate with the virtue of the different elements? How do I shift my nonverbal communications intentionally, so that I can more effectively offer to my client whatever helps them thrive? We recognize that thriving by the easing of the client's body and the coming into physical rapport: breathing, ease, increased vitality.

We're always communicating, even when we're not speaking. There's a message conveyed, other than the verbal content, all the time- whether it is deliberate or not. Don't kid yourself, you're always giving a message... So why not make it an intentionally supportive healing message for that client?

WATER

Water is about the transformation of Virtue from Fear to Wisdom, via reassurance. What is Fear, what is wisdom, what is reassurance? They are physical states, and so to understand them, we need to work through the body. Find your body. Find your willingness to be in your body. Anchoring.

Pretend you're stupid. But nice. Sort of like a panda bear. They don't have a computer running up there. Radiant panda bear. Excessively deployed Intelligence can make us feel separate from humanity due to an endless buzzing in the head. Settle. Sink into your bones.

Fear. Fear has a lot to do with the unknown. It's the acute awareness of the unknown in its raw state. People who do not have a significant Water element tend to be happy to ignore what they don't know. "Hey, if I don't know, it doesn't matter."

A person who has strong Water in their constitution can't help but be aware, all the time, of just how much they don't know. Where is your family? How are they? What's happening in your liver? We don't know what's going on in our own bodies! We don't know what's going on in our best friend's mind. There are so many areas of unknown. It is important, and we don't know. A Water person can't help but be aware of that critical unknown. This awareness is what gives rise to the entry level for the virtue of Wisdom, namely Fear: a gut feeling of being quite aware of how much I don't know, that matters.

How Fear manifests can be incredibly various- and these are the various disharmonies of the Water element. I can get all revved up and say "Oh my gosh, I have to be incredibly smart, incredibly clever, and never be caught without my utility belt on, so that no matter what the universe throws my way, I will have an acupuncture point for it." This can lead to Yin deficiency because it keeps us on turbo-overdrive.

Or, other kinds of fear, particularly a "collapsing" fear, can lead to Kidney Yang deficiency: "I'm doomed, I'm doomed, doomed!" Doom gives us a sense of certainty. 'I'm doomed' can, paradoxically, be a relief, because it's a known, it's an escape from the endless uncertainty. Being doomed you don't have to worry about the unknown possibilities... But it leads to sinking, collapsing, not even trying, being frozen.

I don't do this with every client, but this was one very doomed Water type who I called "Mr. Know-it All". I'd say to him, ranting sarcastically, "You know everything. You know everything there is to know. You know you're doomed. You know everything about the entire universe, all the possibilities, everything that could happen in your life, and you're sure. Doom."

"Okay" he said, "I don't know everything. Maybe... I only might be doomed."

"Aha!"

Once you only might be doomed, it's really different. We're back in the realm of possibility.

There are many ways to go into Fear, which may be differentially diagnosed. What they all have in common is all Fear is the entry level to Wisdom. What is Wisdom? Wisdom is not Knowledge. From the *Tao de Ching* "Every day in pursuit of the Tao, something is let go." The character for Wisdom can also be translated as Know-how. Competence. Mastery. Life confidence. Wisdom is knowing what to do when nobody knows what to do. Like when your 15 year old is stealing cars- nobody knows what to do. There isn't a body of knowledge for that. That's when you seek out a wise person, probably an older person who's been through something like this. They will have listened to life enough that they're able to go into the deep listening that allows us to catch things that we wouldn't catch if we were afraid to sit in the dark for a long time and be with the unknown....

This is the beginning of Wisdom.

There's a way in which Wisdom is the perpetual beginner's mind of the Master. It's the ability to, in any situation, (even one you've known for years), to be simultaneously equally aware of all you don't know. In fact, that's where the help comes from. "I don't know" at first gives rise to terror. Entry to the Virtue is Fear. The people who know what they don't know are the fearful ones. But, over time, they get practice with not knowing, and settling into it, and become Life's Deep Listeners. The ones who are unafraid of not knowing. And so, they stay in the not knowing for longer. This leads to a beginner's mind, an absence of prejudice. From not knowing comes an openness that is the beginning stages of Wisdom. It's by living in this state of not knowing that we hear, see, and pick up on the fine nuances that would be completely glossed over if all we were seeing was what we know. Wisdom is not being blind to what you know; it's also being open to what you don't know at the same time, and being comfortable in that not knowing.

How do we assist somebody who's in the active state of Fear, which is potentially a physiologically very damaging state? This is why it concerns us. Not because they're unhappy, not because they don't like it, and are uncomfortable, but because we're medical workers. They're in a physiologically damaging chronic state. We're not therapists; it's not about talking, talking. We want to help them shift out of a physiologically damaging state into experiencing the exact same emotion, (because they've likely got good reasons for it), but in such a way that it becomes a healing journey. In this way Fear becomes not only no longer damage but actually the path of Sage-hood. This shift also has profound physiological consequences. Again, as medical workers, this is why we do it.

The 5 Element lore is that the proper healing response to Fear on the part of the practitioner is to give reassurance. Now, I've seen a lot of bullshit symptomatic crap reassurance go down. For example, when I was 13 years old, my mother got what was diagnosed as an inner ear infection. I had to spend my whole Christmas vacation taking care of her. My first day back at school, she said, "Try to have a good day. See you back home." I was sick and tired of taking care of my mom. I stayed late after school. Got back home just as the ambulance was driving away. She was dead on arrival from an aneurysm. I didn't know that yet. I just knew an ambulance drove away, and there was blood all over the bedroom.

I can't tell you how many relatives, as we waited for the call from the hospital, said "It'll be okay. It'll be all right".

Now nobody's getting over me with any bullshit reassurance any more. Nobody's going to tell me it's gonna be 'all right'. Nobody's going to get between me and the unknown anymore. That's not healing. That's not reassurance. That's bullshit.

Cheap reassurance is a symptomatic treatment of fear: "Stop being aware of the unknown. Change it to a certainty. Now you won't have to face the unknown anymore." Is this helpful? Or, is this treating the symptom, hoping it goes away? It's gonna come back. Maybe it worked for a moment. You gave them certainty, just for a moment. If you're convincing enough, authoritative enough, sound enough like God, with a deep booming resonant Water voice. ..

How's this for reassurance: The oil light comes on. Snip

the wire to the oil light. "You're all better! See?"

Telling me the words- 'it'll be okay' or 'it's your karma' is worse than useless. What I need is a physiological shift, not a shift in my beliefs. Because I can change my head, but if I'm not changing the thing inside me that's humming like a refrigerator because my adrenals won't drop their idle, then it hasn't actually helped on the level of shifting physiology, which is what we're in the business of doing. Otherwise, we have no business messing with somebody's emotions. Our sole intent in working with someone's psycho-spiritual material is to make shifts from physiologically harmful ways of having our emotions to physiologically beneficial ways of having those same emotions. That's how we know we're not meddlers. That's where we get the nerve: because of our responsibility to the client's body.

So, what do we need to do? The words that accompany the message may be useful for the mind. I'm trained by veterinarians. I'm interested in the communication with other people's bodies, and I'm interested in what inarticulate people can do to offer reassurance. And that has a lot to do with our body language.

The way a veterinarian communicates reassurance has a lot to do with physical density. Being in our bodies in a dense way, and giving your chair a lot to hold up. So, let your pelvis be a bowling ball. Be the base of a pyramid. Offer the view from the bottom of the fish tank. The bottom of the ocean.

Making the dark be an acceptable place to be.

Settle, and be able to start working from the place that is

infinite. What I don't know is infinite. What I don't know will always be infinite- there's no changing that. ...So, can I sit at the bottom of the ocean, welcoming what I don't know, and sitting, solid, communicating to the client the solidness of the chair, the solidness of what is contained within us.

Leon Hammer did this for me most profoundly. It was like the antidote to that nonsense about my mother being 'all right' which sort of ripped my Kidney meridian for awhile. I was in my early 20's, I was very ill, I was passing out for no known reason, could not be revived for 4 or 5 minutes at a time, nobody could find anything wrong. Leon was a friend of mine and he was looking into my case and was going to help me, wanted to.

I said to him, "Leon, am I going to make it?"

Completely from this embrace and this solidness, he looked at me and he said, "I don't know". And, in that moment, I could feel that feeling of 'everything *is* going to be all right.' And not because I know what's going to happen. But because within what happens is what was going to happen. That this is the way the ocean is flowing. This is the way life is moving. And I'm able to settle in that. And the known is that Leon is here with me right now and I am here right now, and I am what I am. Sometimes in a situation, I am the only known factor, but that's something. And, in fact, it's a very big something.

We are always functioning with that 50/50, known and unknown. And, the unknown may be everything outside of us. And part of what's inside of us. But, there's also, this

'I am this.' And, that's what I'm going to live from, is what I am. So, in some sense, there's an inevitability to it. What I'm going to do, if it's going to be successful by any standard, especially by the Tao's standard, but what I'm going to do is what *I* would do. I can try doing what my first grade teacher would have done, what my father would have done, what my lawyer would have done, what my ex-wife would have done, what my best friend would have done, and that's never going to be our ace. Our best possible shot is to do what *we* would do, because this is our life, and we got into this situation.

And yet, when we're in that state of fear, not yet moved to wisdom, we're usually in that post-school state- we go to school to find out that doing it our way is wrong. The minute we write a paper and get a B minus, we get the message that being authentically who we are is not good enough. And then we either become yin deficient, by trying, trying, trying to be the smartest, or become Yang deficient by getting doomed, doomed, doomed and discouraged.

And, what we're doing with our reassurance: it's a body language of sinking down. The voice sinks down, the sound is a groan, but it's a powerful groan, it's the groan of the bottom of the ocean. The groan of the silence that contains all noise, that kind of deep, holding sound. And then, whatever it is that we're saying to the client, what we're really saying to the client is: there's an entire ocean of Tao supporting you. Just like this chair is supporting me. We are supported. You are not doing this on your own. The unknown is your resource. It's just an unknown resource. And you are the other resource.

And, whatever words we find, we may find words like, "How about 3:00 on Thursday?", but do you hear what I mean about, you can say "How about 3:00 on Thursday?", and the person can suddenly feel that the bottom that has dropped out is solid again. "Okay, time to get up on the treatment table". There is a bottom to this ocean, you will not drown in your life. As a healing, this is the new possibility. We're making space, we're bringing in light, and we're bringing in, through body language and voice, the sound, not necessarily the words, because people can argue with words, we're just bringing in the awareness of a new possibility. The possibility that the bottom will hold. The possibility that the unknown bears us forward. It's not just that the unknown will hurt us. It also holds us. And there is what we do know. What I am.

It really takes being down in the gritty with somebody. People really appreciate you're lending your body to their cause. And coming down and not just saying it up here, but coming down to where their body is at. And under it. You're getting under them, with strength, with vitality. Speaking with that voice. Like if Darth Vader were a good guy. That kind of voice.

You don't have to try to do anything. This is all 'cup runneth over' business. All we are doing is being in the reassurance. Actually anchoring in it.

People will say anything. What is the sound? Not the words.

WOOD

Anger. What is anger? Anger is the trembling and starting of the Liver meridian. Like when you start the car. The arousing tumult of Spring which can be pathological. Can be a physiologically damaging state. There are many kinds of anger - these are all different patterns of disharmony of Wood- all kinds of bad moods- and the Virtue within them. But all of them have in common this trembling and starting quality that has to do with ...

One of the ways to understand an element is to understand it's what it's between. It's between Water and Fire. Think of it as an acute potential of Water not manifesting fast enough. I'm trying to move from potential to manifestation and "This is in my Way!!"

Which acknowledges an insight. Anger acknowledges the possibility of progress. Anger requires a progressive eye. You've got to think there's something wrong before you fix it. It's the person who noticed there was a problem.... It takes a visionary to get angry. ...

Wood is the element of heroes. Earth helps take care of you while you're small and weak. But this is more like-- 'I'm big and strong. I can do it. Let's go.' Action. Going to move the log out of the road. When anger is healthy anger it moves from arousal to Constructiveness.

From seeing a problem to solving it, for the good of humanity. This is what's meant by Benevolence.

Why I tend to be focused on Virtue- it makes my day

so much less depressing. I'm surrounded all day by future Sages. ...To see in someone's Rage the seeds of Heroism.

How do we get from Anger to Constructiveness? The 5 Element lore is you give a Wood person Direction. Just as with Reassurance, there are symptomatic 'fixes', and what I see people doing instead of giving Direction is giving 'directions': Do this.

What's needed is progressive movement. Telling somebody what to do will work temporarily. What we're really wanting for a person is they develop inside themselves a sense of direction. What does that mean? A number of different things.

A statement about the nature of life: I would say that plants are alive and that rocks are not alive. Rocks don't have babies, and you can't kill them. Are we okay with this distinction?

Trees are alive. Fire is not alive. Water is not alive. Earth is not alive.

The scientific definition of aliveness includes the capacity to reproduce.

Wood has the distinction of being the only Alive one. One of the qualities of aliveness is the capacity for Growth. How alive are we? Children seem so very alive. What do we mean by that? It's rapidly growing. We see the aliveness of it in its rapid growth.

Anger. Constructiveness. It's not just any movement. It's growth. Evolution. To progress. This kind of growth. Self-organized direction, coming out to manifest. Direction of Wood is from Water to Fire. From potential to manifestation. This has something to do with whether the anger is constructive. Is this anger moving potential towards manifestation? That sense of progress, of movement. Or is this anger not moving any potential whatsoever toward manifestation? That is not constructiveness. That's the kind of anger that will be physiologically problematic. That is not causing more potential to come into manifestation.

The movement from Water to Fire, the movement from Dark to Light, the movement from Root to Sun that plants have an unerring sense of direction. Plants always grow towards the light. That's what they do. From the dark. We also grow from the struggles, from the challenges, from the difficulties. Healthy Wood grows from the dark toward the light.

Real plants in nature never lose their sense of direction. Those sunflowers, all day long, following the light. But we, in our anger, lose our sense of direction of moving toward the Light, toward the Heart, the sun within ourselves. One minute you're a nice guy, next minute, somebody takes your parking spot...Where'd that Heart go? And where's all that energy of progress going? Towards the Heart? Towards the light? Or, did we just do a hairpin turn? From what we said our goals are, what our life is about?

This is what we are giving. From minor tick-off to something that will benefit humanity. Why? One, I can't think of anything better to do, but Two- because of the physiological shift in the person...This is not morality speaking. It works morally. I'm glad that the process of making this shift also has the side-effect of making people better citizens. But, we're doing it out of medical responsibility, not moral 'You should be like this". This is an important distinction. We have no business trying to advocate saintliness and heroism in our people.

It is, however, our business, to help people work with their anger in such a way that it will be physiologically beneficial to them rather than destructive to them. By helping them create a sense of direction. Is this working towards the Heart? Or, is this actually turning your Heart into a dismal dark place? Are you moving toward the light?

This one I'll ask verbally: "Are you willing to be constructive about this?" Because that will often stop people in their tracks a bit. It's a rare person who's angry- if the anger really is a Wood issue- that says 'No, I don't want to be constructive."

During spring day, everything's moving all over the place. During spring night, everything goes into a crouch. Shout is the sound of 'call to action'- it says, "on your mark, get set..."

To live with hope in a more aroused state, to be in the plotting and planning and configuring. Vision- You have no idea what's around the corner. When we lose hope, this is what closes. We have hope first, and vision second. We may be in a valley of our life. If you're in a valley, you're not going to have vision. And yet, we shut, we lose hope, collapse in it, if we lose hope. Part of our responsibility as a practitioner is to keep hope alive, because after five years in a dead-end job, the feeling is different from "I don't know yet, but when the possibility comes, when the vision comes..."

When Harriet Tubman finally comes and says, "Come on up, I've got a lifeline", will they have a liver like a Brillo pad and a Gall Bladder full of liquid Drano and crushed hopes. Or will they say, Okay, I've been looking for this?"

We don't really know what's going to happen out there. Our responsibility is physiology and that means growth. Within this situation, how can this person grow?

I try not to talk that much. The body language is the most important part of getting people up and moving, but I will ask questions about constructiveness and I will ask questions about growth.

Most people kind of think that growth is for plants, or kids. There's a whole lot of anger that wouldn't be happening in the first place if we greeted a hassle as "another fucking growth opportunity". If we took that more seriously-the obstacle makes this arousal in us. Okay: life is signaling growth. Usually what happens is something out there gets our attention and we think it should change. It stinks. It's stupid. It should change, not me grow. Or if what's happening out there is fine with me, why should I change? This sets a Wood Element up for a certain amount of indignation at most, if not all times. What can you get out of this? How can you become stronger?

Constructiveness. What I find is that not all anger is actually anger. Of all the emotions, anger is the emotion least likely to actually be anger. Anger is where we go when we don't want to feel what we actually feel because it makes us feel too passive, so we go into action mode rather than feeling mode. When actually it's something else entirely.

Worseley says no anger is worse than an Earth person who thinks their needs are not being met because nobody cares about their needs. If they don't want to be constructive, If they're a Wood person, constructiveness feels great because constructiveness gives them a place to go. But if it's actually "You don't care about me...", if self-pity and helplessness are at the bottom of it, then treating Wood is not going to help. Anger could be Earth. Anger could be Fear. Road rage is actually terror- adrenaline with nowhere to go. I don't want to feel the Fear. They don't want to be constructive, they want to kill or be killed. And it's actually reassurance, that deep, deep steadiness that will allow them to amp back down.

Anger also can be a cover for Fire- "You don't love me". People want to feel loved all of the time. Affirmation and connection.

When I'm in "machine mode", Fire people get very upset. This is a "Do you love me?" problem. If you don't love me, I hate you. It feels like a death to not be loved, especially for a Fire person.

Metal anger is- "you have offended my honor, and one of us must die". This is the attempt not to feel grief.

Find your body. Let's do some Liver Blood tonification.

Come and sit inside your own skin, and feel the ocean inside your own skin. There are many aspects to that ocean, but all of it is yours. You're sitting in a jacuzzi of yourself, and feeling the whole ocean move, and there are many different portions to this ocean, starting with the deep dark Shu di Huang Rehmannia depths of the ocean. This is my inner world. This is the flavor of myself, in the depth of my ocean. Bai Shao Peony, the big reservoir of the Blood, it's a big place in here. You can let it be bigger, and even fuller. And the Dang Gui of the ocean of the Blood, the place where the fishes live. Starts to come up to the chest level, there are emotions inside of me. I'm so full of fish- life, feeling all that moves in my Blood. All that I've taken in today, all my responses to it, all the way out to the edges of my skin, like Chuan Xiong, it moves, up to the waves, from the very depths of my ocean inside to the skin, full. And taste your ocean. It's a unique flavor. Not only is it unique to you, it's unique to this moment, so taste it, your own Blood., your own ocean, your own inner experience of yourself.

If you were a tea, taste how you'd taste if you were made with two tea-bags instead of one. A rich infusion. Not just a tea. A steep infusion of what I feel like, taste like. And from this fullness, notice that there's a world outside of your skin, too. But, see if you can keep it at least 50/50. Half of my awareness is of my inner world, half of my awareness is of the outer world.

Fairly often, mostly with women but it happens with men also, Blood deficient men, we get so aware of the outer world that we lose our awareness of our inner world. Blood deficiency is usually the feeling of- in a one on one confrontation, we feel outnumbered. We feel small on the inside, because we're not fully filling and feeling our own ocean.

We are fully half of any experience we are in. We are fully half of any situation. It's inside of your skin.

Here's a Bai Shao Peony story. Changed my life. I did a Bradley birth class before my son was born, and one of the other women in the class was a very tall black martial artist, children's abuse rights attorney. You can just imagine the hostility that comes from short, white lawyers, what that woman works with, Wood Constitution. She had the birth plan worked out with this doctor, she was going to have this natural birth. She was at this hospital because of some backup plans she wanted because of some family medical history.

Gets to the hospital in advanced labor, the doctor takes the birth plan and rips it up in front of her and says, "We're doing it my way".

She looks at the doctor and says, "Nope", and goes back to the waiting room, does almost all of her labor in the waiting room, finally comes and says, "Okay, I'm ready to give birth now". They immediately try to start hooking her up to a million monitors, somebody says, "Your water hasn't burst yet, we're going to burst it", basically for the next period of time until the baby was out, there was not a five minute period that she was not saying no to somebody.

She's telling me this story later with this little baby in her arms, and I'm getting so tense, so angry, muscle cramped in victim consciousness. Finally, it dawned on me that she wasn't looking angry. I said to her, "Aren't you furious at that doctor". She said, "This was my first birth, I wasn't going to let some doctor ruin my first birth."

Oh man. On so many levels, I didn't want to hear that. That woman was not outnumbered by what was going on outside of her because she had so much Blood, so much self-esteem, so much fullness of her own internal ocean that she was half of the situation, the good half. And she was able to hold her own. And suddenly, my entire life had to be revised. Because every single place there was this victim....

When I was 15 years old, my father wouldn't let me be alone with anyone who was male, ever, which put a serious cramp in my conversations with male friends. I had been so angry , and cramped about that, and all these other things my parents did.

She would've just had whatever conversations she was going to have. Blood deficient, angry victim, defensive, what is defensiveness? It's a muscle cramp. I'm already outnumbered, and you haven't even hit me.

Martin Luther King, there's Liver Blood for you. No victimhood; even when there has been a clear trespass, Liver Blood is the ability to respond from fullness of self-esteem.

Glossary of Chinese Medicine Terms

Yin- literally- the shady side of the hill- the moist, cool, calm, receptive, and stereotypically feminine principle

Yang- literally the sunny side of a hill- the warm, active, initiating, fiery, stereotypically masculine principle

Qi- the animating force within or behind all life forms

Tai Chi Chuan- a meditative martial art form, practiced for its health benefits (including contribution to longevity) and for self defense

Qi Gong- Internal and physical methods of "energy cultivation", used for both preventative and curative purposes in Traditional Chinese Medicine.

Shen- Spirit, awareness, consciousness

Moxibustion- a traditional Chinese technique involving the burning of dried mugwort (a spongy, aromatic plant) near or occasionally on the patient's skin. The purpose of moxibustion is to move the qi, warm and strengthen the Blood, and maintain one's health.

Dan tian- Literal translation: "elixir field". An important focal point for internal meditative techniques. Usually refers to the physical center of gravity, located in the abdomen three fingers below the navel, and two finger widths behind the navel.

NOTES

(1) Angell, Marcia: "The Epidemic of Mental Illness: Why?" New York Review of Books, June, 2011

(2) Whitaker, Robert, Anatomy of an Epidemic: Magic Bullets, Psychiatric Drugs, and the Astonishing Rise of Mental Illness in America, Crown Publishers, New York: 2010.

(3) Cooper, Arnie: Christopher Lane On What's Wrong with Modern Psychiatry The Sun, Chapel Hill, NC, March, 2012

(4) Lewis, Amini and Lannon, *A General Theory of Love*, New York: Random House, 2000, pp. 176-190

(5) Wu J, Yeung, AS, Schnyer R, Wang, Y, Mischoulon, D "Acupuncture for depression: a review of clinical applications". [Journal Article] *Can J Psychiatry* 2012 Jul; 57(7):397-405.

(6) Erickson, Milton and Rosen, Sidney (ed.), *My Voice Will Go With You: The Teaching Tales of Milton H. Erickson* , New York: WW Norton, 1982.

(7) Lipinski, Jed, "Anatomy of an Epidemic- the Hidden Damage of Psychiatric Drugs", April, 2010, Salon. com

(8) Shen Nong Ben Cao Jing (Divine Husbandman's Classic of Materia Medica) Han Dynasty (206 B.C.-220 A.D.) considered the earliest pharmacopeia in China.

(9) Thea Elijah, "the Perennial Medicine"
http://www.perennialmedicine.com/ArticlesandTranscripts.html
pp. 1, 2

Acknowledgments

I'm grateful to the people who took the time to read part or all of my manuscript, and to tell me ways they could imagine I might make it better:

David Spero, Janet Rode Siegel, Thea Elijah, Stephen Cowan, Elaine Wolf Komarow, Stacy Snyder, Jenny Wood, David Schwartz, Martine Bellen, Melissa Everett, Peter Eckman, Z'ev Rosenberg, Deborah Lemont, and Andrew Seubert.

I'm delighted to be able to include articles by Stephen Cowan, MD, Thea Elijah, L.Ac., and Heiner Fruehauf, PhD as Appendices.

Thanks to Michael Broffman for introducing me to the world of Chinese medicine, and for suggesting I re-read and write about *Dream of the Red Chamber*.

BIBLIOGRAPHY

Hammer, Leon, *Dragon Rises, Red Bird Flies: Psychology and Chinese Medicine*, Barrytown, NY: Station Hill Press, 1990.

Lewis, Amini, and Lannon, *A General Theory of Love*, New York: Random House, 2000.

Erickson, Milton and Rosen, Sidney (ed.), *My Voice Will Go With You: The Teaching Tales of Milton H. Erickson* , New York: WW Norton, 1982.

Angell, Marcia: "The Epidemic of Mental Illness: Why?" New York Review of Books, June, 2011

Whitaker, Robert, *Anatomy of an Epidemic: Magic Bullets, Psychiatric Drugs, and the Astonishing Rise of Mental Illness in America*, New York: Crown Publishers, 2010.

Cooper, Arnie: *Christopher Lane On What's Wrong with Modern Psychiatry* **The Sun**, Chapel Hill, NC, March, 2012

Michael T Greenwood, MD, "Acupuncture And Evidence-Based Medicine: A Philosophical Critique", *Medical Acupuncture Online Journal* , Volume 13,   No. 2, Article 4.

Roger Jahnke, OMD, Linda Larkey, PhD; Carol Rogers, APRN-BC, CNOR, PhD; Jennifer Etnier, PhD; Fang Lin, MS, "A Comprehensive Review of health Benefits of Qigong and Tai Chi", 2010

Wu J, Yeung AS; Schnyer, R; Wang, Y; Mischoulon, D Acupuncture for depression: a review of clinical applications. [Journal Article] Can J Psychiatry 2012 Jul; 57(7):397-405

Michael Broffman, L.Ac. and Michael McCulloch, MPH, L.Ac., "Integrative Traditional Chinese Medicine and Chemotherapy: Survival Data in Node-Positive and Metastatic Breast Cancer" in San Francisco Medicine: Journal of the San Francisco Medical Society, November-December, 2001

Tsao Hsueh-chin, Dream of the Red Chamber, first published 1791, translated and abridged by Wang Chi-Chen, 1929, published by Anchor, 1958.

CPSIA information can be obtained at www.ICGtesting.com
Printed in the USA
LVOW08s0819220316

480220LV00005B/171/P